FACE THE FACTS

• A centuries-old folk remedy called Valerian—proven effective against numerous medical complaints—is available virtually anywhere in the world . . . except the United States!

• In California, a three-month supply of Tenormin and Dyazide (hypertension), Mevocor (high cholesterol), and Tagamet (ulcers) costs $325. Just over the border in Mexico, it's almost $200 less!

• Desperately ill AIDS patients are forced to travel to foreign countries for treatments that could have been available in the U.S. long ago!

• It would not be financially profitable for American drug manufacturers to produce the medicines used for treating Tourette's syndrome, Lou Gehrig's disease and other rare ailments . . . so they don't!

Now, at last, it's easy to order these and a long list of other pharmaceuticals from abroad. This unique and essential handbook tells you how!

How To Buy Almost Any Drug *Legally* Without A Prescription

JAMES H. JOHNSON, Ph.D.

AVON BOOKS NEW YORK

HOW TO BUY ALMOST ANY DRUG LEGALLY WITHOUT A PRESCRIPTION is an original publication of Avon Books. This work has never before appeared in book form.

Before using any medication, it is strongly recommended that you first consult your physician. People with diagnosed health conditions should seek treatment under the guidance and supervision of a physician and licensed pharmacist. Because each person's tolerance level for medications differs, it is especially important that a physician monitor such conditions and that you follow recommendations to take the proper medication in the proper amount to most effectively treat that condition. No one should commence taking any drugs without the recommendation of a physician.

This book was thoroughly researched and reflects at press time the most current information regarding the medications included and how to mail-order them. Neither the publisher nor the author takes responsibility for addresses, phone numbers, or prices that may have changed without notification.

AVON BOOKS
A division of
The Hearst Corporation
1350 Avenue of the Americas
New York, New York 10019

Copyright © 1990 by James H. Johnson
Published by arrangement with the author
Library of Congress Catalog Card Number: 90-93177
ISBN: 0-380-76033-9

Library of Congress Cataloging in Publication Data:

Johnson, James H.
    How to buy almost any drug legally without a prescription / James H. Johnson.
      p.   cm.
    Includes bibliographical references (p.   ) and index.
1. Pharmaceutical policy—United States.   2. United States. Food and Drug Administration.   3. Drugs—United States—Purchasing.
4. Mail-order business—Directories.   I. Title.
RA401.A3J64   1990
362.1'782'0973-dc20
                                                            90-93177
                                                            CIP

First Avon Books Printing: December 1990

AVON TRADEMARK REG. U.S. PAT. OFF. AND IN OTHER COUNTRIES, MARCA REGISTRADA, HECHO EN CANADA

Printed in Canada

UNV 10 9 8 7 6 5 4 3 2

Acknowledgments

It is important for me to mention that along the way of writing this book I received a great deal of assistance from numerous individuals within the FDA who are deeply concerned about America's health care crisis, as well as from officials of the DEA, and from embassies and consulates around the world. Staff members at Project Inform and at the *AIDS Treatment News*, both located in San Francisco, all went out of their way to help me. To name all of these people and thank them would be impossible.

There are two people, however, who deserve special thanks. Linda Boroff did much of the actual research and draft writing for this book. Its completion would have been impossible without her relentless energies. Dr. Kathy Johnson did exceptional work in editing the final manuscript.

Contents

Preface

This book began one December morning in 1988 when I read an article in the *San Francisco Chronicle* with the headline, "FDA Allows Mail-Order of Foreign Drugs."

As a former professor at two different medical schools, I was in shock that the Food and Drug Administration (FDA) would even think of an idea so radical. I believed, like most other Americans, that we should always "check with our physician first" regarding anything medical or pharmaceutical.

I don't know exactly why I believed this so strongly. Maybe because I had heard it repeated by physicians over and over again in the media. Certainly this belief is unique to the US public, as it is not shared in most other countries.

Article of faith or not, my belief began to crumble as I thought about what I read. Why, I wondered, would a conservative medical bastion like the FDA change its rules to allow Americans to buy almost any legal drug (except controlled substances such as Valium, Librium, etc.) without a prescription by mail order from another country?

Being a scientist at heart, I had to check this out. So I picked up the phone and called the FDA. First, I spoke with the public relations people who had been designated to talk to the public about this decision. After getting only minimal information, I asked to speak directly to key officials.

According to certain FDA employees, the new policy

resulted from pressure by various AIDS groups. And while many of these FDA employees privately disagreed with the change, they were unanimous in admitting that what was being called a "trial policy" by the public relations people, was in reality, here to stay.

How could this change have come about? The answer was simpler than I ever imagined. By instituting this new policy, the FDA's key decision makers were acknowledging that something was seriously wrong with the way our medical system serves the public.

The present system, although very diligent, was painfully slow in the approval of new treatments. As the reporters at *Business Week* stated on February 19, 1990: "Historically, the FDA has been about as swift and adventurous as an arthritic turtle."

The effects of this slowness began to be realized by the FDA as AIDS spread through the population. Those who had AIDS were furious as they faced their own imminent deaths while the government prevented them access to drugs that could save their lives, insisting that these drugs go through the standard five- to eight-year FDA approval process.

Try as the medical community might, there was no denying the magnitude of the AIDS crisis. While estimates vary greatly, it is thought that between 20,000 and 40,000 Americans died of AIDS during 1989 alone. Estimates of the cumulative number of AIDS-related deaths in the United States through middle 1990 are in excess of 81,000. According to the US Public Health Service, 179,000 people will have died from AIDS by the end of 1991.

And these figures are growing at an alarming rate. John S. James, publisher of the *AIDS Treatment News*, estimates that the total number of AIDS deaths doubles every eighteen months. If this estimate is correct, it means that a total of 716,000 people will have died from AIDS by the end of 1994 if new treatments aren't found and brought to market quickly.

It was the awful realization of these grim facts that brought about the revolution. Led by FDA commissioner Frank Young, agency officials saw no alternative but to make policy changes that would upset one of the most powerful political lobbies in the United States: the American Medical Association (AMA).

Young knew that he was taking a huge personal risk. He is quoted as saying, "When I became commissioner, they told me: 'Whatever you do, remember that only one person got an award at the FDA—and that was for doing nothing.' "

The AMA would surely oppose any change that would lessen physician control over the medical process, and the AMA was not a pleasant group to fight with. Despite the prospect of drawing fire, in Young's view, America's health care problems were so big that changes had to be made even if it meant great personal sacrifice. As could be expected, he lost his commissioner's job less than a year after this decision.

In spite of Young's efforts, the FDA is clearly to blame for many of the problems in the current health system. According to an industry spokesman, pharmaceutical manufacturers are unable to develop new treatments for many ailments because the cost of obtaining FDA approval is too high and the expected returns too low. Even worse, the red tape involved in obtaining FDA approval is so great that the process takes years to complete and causes many of the brightest scientists to choose different fields of endeavor.

Even with the reams of press releases coming from the AMA, the pharmaceutical manufacturers, and the FDA, the last real breakthrough drug released in America was the Salk polio vaccine. And that was decades ago!

The fact of the matter is that over the years the FDA has been turned into an agency whose major function has been to slow progress in the development of new treatments. Concerns for public safety have turned obsessive and counterproductive.

And it took the spread of AIDS to make clear to most Americans the inability of the FDA to act quickly. We all were forced to witness Rock Hudson and other AIDS victims traveling to foreign countries to obtain treatments for their illness—treatments that were not "approved" in the US.

What was started as a system designed for the good of the people has evolved into a bureaucratic nightmare and a financial albatross that is strangling the very people it was designed to help.

When I began to recognize that, like our automobile industry, our medical-pharmaceutical industry isn't making it in the modern age, I decided to write this book. Americans deserve better health care than they are getting. And if they are unable to obtain help from the medical or pharmaceutical communities, then they should be able to go elsewhere to get what they need.

Introduction

Before even thinking about importing drugs from other countries you have to understand our medical-pharmaceutical system and be aware of how it came about.

While I have many quarrels with our current system, I am also well aware that much of it evolved for reasons that are entirely sensible. Taking poorly tested drugs can have terrible consequences for people, so there needs to be a proper amount of testing before any new drug is released for use in the general population.

I believe that in most cases, people should only buy and use tested, FDA-approved medications. As can be seen in the following pages, tragedy has often resulted when proper testing has not taken place.

But I also believe that people should keep in mind that other countries have drug-approval processes of their own. They usually have testing agencies that are both skilled and informed. And in most cases these foreign drug-approval agencies take much less time than the FDA. If that worries you, remind yourself that people live longer in many of these countries than they do in the US.

The problem in America is that approval, non-approval, or even an outright ban by the FDA is not necessarily synonymous with careful testing.

You have to be an informed consumer to know when you are getting the truth from the FDA and when to pay attention to its pronouncements. I hold this belief because I know that the FDA has a strong political side to its "testing."

Take, for example, the FDA import alert that was released in September 1988 that bans the import of mifepristone (RU 486) as unsafe. This is the so-called "abortion pill" that has been used successfully for several years in France as a relatively safe, easy way to bring about an abortion in the early stages of pregnancy.

A recent study reported in the *New England Journal of Medicine* (March 1990), based on 2115 women who used RU 486 to induce abortions, showed that 96 percent had no more side effects than with conventional procedures. In this study only a small percentage of women even experienced minor side effects such as nausea, vomiting, dizziness, abdominal pain, or excessive bleeding.

RU 486 resulted in successful abortions for 2052 of these women. The drug only failed to bring about an abortion for twenty out of this entire group. An additional forty-three of these women experienced only partial abortions and then had to undergo standard surgical procedures.

It should be especially noted that not one of the 2115 subjects died in the process. Compared with the results of surgical abortion, this is simply amazing.

One obstetrician, Charles Plow, M.D., of Anaheim, California, has been quoted in the *San Francisco Chronicle* of March 7, 1990 as saying that use of the pill, if it were approved by the FDA, would result in a reduction of thousands of deaths that are now attributed to surgical abortions.

With huge numbers of women in other parts of the world having used this product safely, most people know that "safety first" is not the real reason behind the FDA's ban of RU 486. This ban is a clear example of the power that groups such as Right to Life have over the FDA. How else could an organization such as the FDA condone the many unnecessary deaths that result in the US each year from its prohibition of RU 486?

And this is not the only case where the FDA seems to

2

be more political than scientific. There are many, many more examples that you will see in the chapters that follow. The FDA is like the little boy who cried wolf too often. You have to know when to take it seriously and when to ignore it.

The only way to find out if the FDA is telling you the truth about the value of any particular medication is to understand how the agency came about and how it operates. Once you have that information, you can put its pronouncements in a context that will allow you to evaluate them properly.

Your own health and safety depend upon your learning to decipher the warnings that come from the FDA. This is true whether you decide to try mail-order importation or not. You need to know whether the FDA pronouncements are "from the heart" and concern safety, from political needs, or from the self-interested lobbying of the pharmaceutical industry and the American Medical Association.

I believe you can learn what you need to know for these purposes from the next few chapters and Appendix II in this book. So read them with serious consideration.

The next thing to be aware of is that the pronouncements of the FDA and the Drug Enforcement Administration (DEA) often have the status of laws. The penalty for ignoring these pronouncements can be severe—a jail sentence. Therefore, pay attention to the chapters that tell explicitly what you cannot import.

This is required reading because FDA rulings do not necessarily follow the dictates of common sense. For example, I bet you would never guess that there is an import alert out (August 20, 1984) against bringing Colgate dental cream with double fluoride into this country.

The remaining chapters in the book will give you an introduction to a number of drugs that appear to be legal to import.

The primary reason for importing a drug is most often

that a drug is cheaper in another country. By ordering from abroad you can save money on most of your current prescription medications.

But another good reason could be that you have a disease or condition that requires a medication that is only available outside the United States. If that is because you have a rare disease, look in chapter IX on orphan drugs. If it is because the FDA has been dragging its feet on approving a drug, look at chapter VIII on investigational drugs.

Or you might be HIV positive and having trouble finding appropriate treatments in your community. (For example, many physicians still don't know about all the drugs that are available outside the United States that can help prolong an AIDS victim's life.)

If you are in this situation, look at chapter X on AIDS. This chapter is as up-to-date as the publication of this book and it has all the necessary underground information on the subject that the FDA isn't talking about. Here you will also find several important sources of information to keep you current in the future as well.

In the appendices of the book I have reproduced copies of all the relevant import alerts that are in effect for those people who want to have more information on the FDA's guidelines. I also provide listings of companies that are willing to sell personal quantities of legal drugs through the mail to American buyers. For your convenience, ordering instructions and sample listings of some of the many available pharmaceuticals are provided along with prices.

WHAT ARE "DRUGS" ANYWAY? WHAT ARE "NEW DRUGS," AND WHAT ARE THE LAWS ABOUT PRESCRIBING THEM?

It is surprising for most people to learn that America has one of the most bureaucratized systems of medicine in the world. There is a law for nearly every aspect of health care in the United States.

Most of these laws are fairly recent, dating from after World War II. Shocking as it may seem, our current system of medical and pharmaceutical practice wasn't handed down to us carved in stone. It was mainly developed one law at a time, during the last fifty years.

So now in 1990 we have a system of medicine which is proscribed by law from the smallest detail to the overall big picture. Very little in this field is left to conjecture. We even have a legal definition of what constitutes a "drug" and what constitutes a "new drug."

The Food, Drug, and Cosmetic Act (21 USC 321) contains a fairly long and intricate definition of the word "drug."

1) The term "drug" means (A) articles recognized in the official United States Pharmacopoeia, official Homeopathic Pharmacopoeia of the United States, or official National Formulary, or any supplement to any of them; and (B) articles intended for use in the diagnosis, cure, mitigation, treatment, or prevention of disease in man or other animals; and (C) articles (other than food) intended to affect the structure or any function of the body of man or other animals; and (D) articles intended for use as a component of any article specified in clause (A), (B), or (C); but it does not include devices or their components, parts or accessories.

This appears to be a straightforward and inclusive definition. In practice, however, a substance may or may not be a drug, depending upon what it is used for. So if water is sold with a therapeutic claim, it would fall within the definition of a drug. The "anticancer drug" Laetrile, which consists basically of ground-up apricot pits, if marketed as a cancer cure, is indeed a drug. Thus, if substances not generally thought of as drugs are "used in the treatment of diseases in man," they are drugs for the purposes of the FDA.

The concept of a "new drug" is also something that the government has wrestled with. Obviously, this is an important distinction for the FDA because it is solely responsible for the approval of all new drugs.

Just because a drug is termed new does not necessarily mean that it is a substance that has never been known before. It might indeed be a very common substance; it is only the *use* for it that is new. By law, the FDA must approve all "new drugs" even though they may actually have been previously approved for a different purpose.

Yet more confusion arises out of who has the authority to prescribe drugs. Common sense would dictate that included within the authority to diagnose and treat a disease would be the authority to prescribe and administer drugs that affect that disease. In most cases that means doctors and dentists. Common sense would also indicate that authority to prescribe would be spelled out clearly in the FDA regulations. But that is not the case. It turns out that who has authority to prescribe is mainly a decision determined by the various state governments, so there is some variation from state to state.

And recently, more and more states have been extending the authority to prescribe drugs to a variety of health professionals other than doctors and dentists. Eighteen states have now extended drug-prescribing authority to physician's assistants and registered nurse practitioners, and two states permit pharmacists to prescribe a limited number of drugs. Three states allow unrestricted prescribing by qualified nurse practitioners.

The legal right to prescribe drugs is more often the result of a battle of professional lobbies at the level of state government. Usually it is a group of nonphysician health care professionals fighting for prescription rights and the AMA fighting against them.

These are generally very serious fights because there is big money involved. Whoever can write prescriptions has a license to become rich. Thanks to government legislation and the FDA, Americans have to pay licensed prescription writers as much as $60 to $80 for simple treatments, ranging from shampoos for head lice to special creams for rashes and pimples.

An interesting side aspect of this is that, in most cases, the legal power to prescribe is usually an "across the board" privilege. So, for example, in most states a dentist can write a prescription for a birth control pill and a physician can write a prescription for fluoride to use for your teeth.

While all of this seems right and natural to most Americans, it is important to be aware that it is seen as idiosyncratic by most of the people in the rest of the world. People in other countries take a much more sensible view. They minimize the amount of government interference in the development of new pharmaceutical treatments. And they don't define almost everything under the sun as a "drug," so it doesn't cost them an arm and a leg to get a new pimple treatment on the market. Consequently, they have a wide range of treatments available for even rare diseases.

People in other countries don't worship at the altar of the medical establishment. (In most places they don't even have a "medical establishment.") They trust themselves for simple (common) drug treatment decisions, and they trust their pharmacist for the rest of their treatment decisions. After all, the pharmacist is the only person in the entire health care spectrum who has actual training on drug usage, drug side effects, and drug interactions. People in other countries designate the physician to serve as the judge for treatment decisions where there is the possibility of addiction or other bad side effects.

For just one example, consider the results of a recent study comparing the outcomes of medical treatment in

Canada versus those in the United States where costs average between 25 and 50 percent higher. Canadian researchers at the University of Manitoba compared outcomes of surgery performed in Manitoba with those performed in New England. Mortality rates differed very little despite the lower Canadian costs. And overall mortality rates for sixty-five-, seventy-five-, and eighty-five-year-old Canadians ranged from 2 to 19 percent lower.

By taking this simple, straightforward view, these people save themselves a lot of money. This also insures that poor people can get treatment as well as rich, so the poor can live longer, healthier lives.

THE HIGH COST OF A PRESCRIPTION IN AMERICA

Some advanced technologies and products get less expensive as time goes by. Back in 1970 a hand-held calculator cost upwards of $100. Today you can wear one on your wrist for as little as $5. But as anyone who has ever had a prescription filled knows, most medicines have not taken that route. Even common antibiotics are still extremely expensive, considering that the technology to produce them has been around for over thirty years.

Today, Americans pay out over $20 billion yearly for prescription drugs. And they pay billions more in doctor's fees just to be allowed to buy these drugs. The tragedy is that many of the people (the elderly, the disabled, and the chronically ill) who need these drugs most can least afford to pay for them. These high costs are a principal cause of why America no longer leads the world in health care and life expectancy.

HOW DID THE AMERICAN PROCESS GO SO WRONG?

You might very well ask who is responsible for the current crisis in America's health care system. The answer is not simple. The problems grew step by step as the federal government passed more and more regulations of the medical and pharmaceutical industries. The United States government passed the Pure Food and Drug Act in 1906, despite the opposition of patent medicine producers. The legislation was drafted largely in response to the muckraking journalists and their crusade against opiate addiction and its consequent vices, which seemed to be on the increase.

The 1906 act required that medicines containing opiates and certain other drugs must state that on the label. Later amendments also required that the quantity of each drug be stated, and that the drug meet official standards of purity and packaging.

However, false statements made by manufacturers were not regulated. Any manufacturer could claim anything he felt appropriate about his product, whether proven true or not. The act did not extend to cosmetics, nor did it grant the government the authority to ban unsafe drugs.

Given such weak legislation, tragedy was inevitable. The first widely documented incident took place in 1937. At that time, a new substance named sulfanilamide was hailed as a "miracle drug," effective against a variety of infections. In the process of creating a cough syrup, one manufacturer decided to mix his sulfa powder with a chemical called diethylene glycol that had a sweet taste and a pleasant light pink color. He was apparently unaware that diethylene glycol was a deadly poison, and because there was inadequate regulation, clinical tests were not performed. Consumers bought the drug, then unknowingly took it or gave it to their children. One hundred seven reported deaths were the result.

Following this, the Food, Drug, and Cosmetic Act of 1938 was passed, requiring testing for safety of all drugs sold in the US. "Safe" was defined as nontoxic when used according to the directions on the label. This new law expanded the meaning of the term "adulteration,"

9

seeking greater guarantees of purity of substances, and extended the law to include cosmetics for the first time.

With the advent of the penicillins during World War II, the pharmaceutical industry grew as never before. Because of the scope and volume of the new antibiotics and the anticipated need for them, the law was expanded once again to cover a requirement for certification of purity and potency.

During these years, the country entered a new era with regard to drugs. A massive group of new medications with functions undreamed of was entering the market. Many of the drugs were of such complex composition and had so many potential adverse reactions or side effects that it was virtually impossible to devise a label that informed the consumer of all pertinent information.

This situation led to the Durham-Humphrey Amendment of 1951, which exempted certain drugs from the labeling requirements. Instead, these drugs were to be dispensed only under the supervision of a medical doctor and were administered under prescription only. Provided with a label stating "Caution: Federal law prohibits dispensing without a prescription" these drugs were now exempt from having to state all of the applicable information on the label. This was the genesis of our present system.

The Thalidomide Disaster of 1962

In 1962 thalidomide, a sleeping pill developed in Europe and widely used abroad, was being studied for release in the United States. Only with the passage of time, however, did the fact become evident that the drug, when taken by a pregnant woman, caused severe deformities in the fetus. Because thalidomide had not yet been brought into the US in marketable quantities, the effect here was proportionately less severe than in Europe, where many children were affected.

For the first time, there was general public realization that drugs could have negative side effects over a longer period of time than was evident under the then-current testing guidelines. The effect of this was that the previous legislation was considered inadequate, and the Kefauver-Harris Amendment of 1962 was passed.

This act was more far-reaching than any previous law. For one thing manufacturers were now required to provide both proof of safety and proof of effectiveness before marketing any new drug. The Good Manufacturing Practices were established as guidelines for quality control. The FDA was to supervise all prescription drugs, while the Federal Trade Commission's jurisdiction was to cover over-the-counter drugs. The amendment additionally established procedures for testing new products. And it established more careful guidelines and reporting procedures.

However, this more careful set of procedures for bringing new drugs to market had the unanticipated effect of being arduous, lengthy, and extremely expensive, even prohibitive—except where there was a widespread demand.

Unintended Consequences of Protective Legislation

Thanks to all the good intentions and well-meant protective measures undertaken by the federal government, the FDA approval process has become unbelievably expensive and time consuming. According to Joseph Dimasi of the Tufts University Center for the Study of Drug Development the average cost today of obtaining FDA approval for a new drug has grown to more than $231 million for a process that now takes an average of twelve years. That is more than double the inflation adjusted cost of just ten years ago! Many experts say that actual cost will double again by the year 2000!

And once a drug is finally available, massive educational, promotional, and advertising expenditures are then required to get doctors to prescribe it. Some drug companies spend over a billion dollars a year on advertising and marketing alone.

The effect of these gargantuan development and marketing costs has actually been quite different from what anyone expected. First, these costs have served to discourage the investigation and development of new and useful drugs, particularly those drugs that might benefit only a small number of people, such as victims of rare diseases. A disease must have a huge incidence rate before it even begins to pay to develop a treatment for it.

Second, the tremendous overall financial commitment involved in the FDA approval process has resulted in skyrocketing pharmaceutical costs. This, in turn, has given the United States the highest medical costs in the world.

Finally, the extended length of time of the FDA approval process has led to a situation where the medical and pharmaceutical communities are no longer able to react on a timely basis to newly emerging diseases.

Take AIDS for example. Even if a new treatment were discovered today, it would take at least six to eight years before the drug could be on the market. Of course, by then it would be far too late for anyone who has the disease today.

WHAT MAKES FDA APPROVAL SUCH A LENGTHY PROCESS?

It is educational to take a brief look at the entire FDA approval process. The amount of time and the procedures that must be followed are almost unbelievably complex and extended.

Because a pharmaceutical company opens itself to

potential lawsuits if the investigation of a new drug is not thorough, the approval process has become so painstaking and cumbersome it is almost a miracle that any new drugs are introduced.

Nevertheless, the potential for profit is so large that countless new drugs are constantly being explored. The drug companies finance their investigations through those few successful drugs that do become superstars. In spite of the millions of dollars spent on research, most new drugs never achieve FDA approval. It is the FDA that is the final decision maker as to which drugs reach the marketplace.

HOW THE FDA IS ORGANIZED

Within the FDA's Center for Drugs and Biologics six divisions are responsible for reviewing all investigational new drugs (INDs). These include the Division of Cardio-Renal Drug Products, the Division of Neuropharmacological Drug Products, the Division of Metabolism and Endocrine Drug Products, the Division of Anti-Infective Drug Products, the Division of Oncology and Radiopharmaceutical Drug Products, and the Division of Surgical-Dental Drug Products.

Each division has numerous medical officers—responsible for reviewing final clinical reports issued by the pharmaceutical companies—as well as biostatisticians, pharmacologists, and chemists. During the course of the drug-approval process the officials of the pharmaceutical companies are constantly meeting with the FDA over all sorts of procedures and test results. The FDA has many guidelines that must be followed and a dizzying number of conditions that must be fulfilled before a drug can even begin being tested.

THE PROCESS OF DRUG TESTING

There is no question that the ultimate test of any drug is its action on human disease. However, prudence dictates that new drugs should be tested first on animals and then introduced to humans. For every one hundred new chemical compounds screened on animals, only one provides activity and safety enough to be considered for clinical testing in man. Of those finally tested on people, less than one in forty (2.5 percent) is ultimately brought to the marketplace.

Because animals are physiologically and biologically different from man, test results cannot be confirmed until humans have used the drug in question. Often many species of animal are tested, starting with rats and mice, proceeding to dogs, cats, and finally to monkeys, before human clinical trials are run.

Next the toxicity of the drug is studied. How effective is it, at what dose is the drug therapeutic, and at what dose toxic? Often the difference is only a thin line. The plan for study of a new drug also includes such issues as dosage range, dosage schedule, duration of treatment, drug interactions, effects on the fetus, adverse reaction evaluations, and many other factors.

What Is a "Clinical Study"?

A clinical study of a drug involves gathering relevant data from which conclusions may be drawn concerning the effectiveness and safety of a particular treatment for a disease or condition. A study team might consist of a chemist, who is fully acquainted with the properties of the drug under study; a pharmacologist or toxicologist, who is responsible for determining how the drug works and at what dosages in man and in animals; a medical clinician or investigator, who is preferably a specialist in the condition or disease being treated; a statistician, who analyzes the data gathered in the course of the trial; and a data-processing expert, who is responsible for recording and storing the information.

Many types of studies are conducted on any drug, and one or all of them may be used to gain information. Among the studies are uncontrolled, parallel and crossover, double-blind and single-blind, random, and more.

In 1987, pharmaceutical firms in the United States spent nearly $2 billion annually in research and development. Needless to say, extensive market research goes along with the development of a drug to ensure that the drug company will find this financial investment worth making.

CHAPTER I

What Is the Government Doing
to Try to Fix This System?

The FDA has made or studied numerous changes in recent years in an effort to improve the medical and pharmaceutical system and to lower costs. To get a better understanding of these attempts, let's look at several that aim to reduce skyrocketing medication costs. Some of them are out there right now, and others just around the corner.

THE GENERIC ALTERNATIVE

The backlash against ever-increasing drug prices was apparent throughout the nineteen eighties and was manifested long before the latest FDA ruling allowing citizens to import certain drugs by mail. Most significantly, widespread public indignation over the high prices of name-brand medications helped bring about the government's decision several years ago to allow generic versions of many drugs onto the market.

What Is a Generic Drug Anyway?

Each drug, as it reaches the clinical testing stage, is assigned a generic name, which is its newly created scientific name. When a patent is issued for a drug, it assures the company that has created it about seventeen years of exclusivity in marketing. Nobody else may sell that specific formula during that period.

During the clinical testing stage, the company creates a brand name for the drug, also known as the proprietary name. For example, chlordiazepoxide has come to be known popularly as Librium. After seventeen years, the drug comes off patent, and companies that can establish their ability to produce the drug according to federal standards, may sell their version of it, under the generic name or under a new brand name they have devised.

Generic versions of popular drugs selling at lower costs brought about some relief from the high prices of brand-name prescription drugs. However, even that adjustment has not been without its drawbacks.

The *New York Times* reported on July 31, 1989 that low-cost generic versions of name-brand pharmaceuticals sometimes have contained substituted materials that actually compromised the drug's effectiveness. Eleven pharmaceutical companies were under investigation for substituting some ingredients in the drugs they offered without obtaining . FDA approval. These substitutions could have altered the chemical stability of the drugs and made them less effective.

The FDA acknowledged that it had reduced its enforcement activities on generics in the wake of its 1984 decision to accelerate procedures with the goal of increasing competition and lowering prices to consumers.

As of June 1990 the scandal has resulted in more than thirteen criminal convictions of generic drug company officials on charges ranging from bribery to racketeering, and the removal from distribution of more than one hundred generic drug products. The end result is likely to be even more FDA regulations and even higher costs for obtaining new drug approval.

OVER-THE-COUNTER DRUGS

The United States is finally beginning to move in the direction that other countries took long ago. It is beginning to dispense entirely with the prescription process for many medications. Only those medications that must be dispensed in a hospital or by the physician are restricted to prescription status.

Self-medication has a long history, reaching back through the centuries to folk medicines. Early American colonists brought many patent medicines with them from England, where royal patents were granted for all manner of remedies. Thus from its very early days, there has been a precedent in the United States for drugs to be available for public purchase and self-directed use.

Currently, self-medication is widespread, with as many as 84 percent of households using some form of over-the-counter (OTC) medication during a thirty-week period. Estimates of the number of over-the-counter drugs in the average household vary between seventeen to twenty-four items. It is thought that 65 to 85 percent of all purchases actually constitute self-care. For example, the availability of even $\frac{1}{2}$ percent hydrocortisone ointment OTC is estimated to have saved the public as much as $1 billion in extra medical and pharmaceutical costs from 1980 to 1982!

Many health experts see OTC drugs as the ultimate solution to the high cost of many prescriptions. Take away the monopoly of drug companies on their particular medication and the prices are bound to fall, just as with any other product that enters the marketplace. Who benefits? Everyone. It's an idea whose time has definitely come. The patient gains, because medicines are cheaper and easier to obtain, and the drug companies themselves stand to benefit as well. Look at what has happened with the several drugs that have changed their status to OTC already.

Until 1985, the drug Advil, whose main ingredient is ibuprofen, was available in the US only as the prescription drug Motrin. The Advil brand name didn't even exist. Now Advil has literally rocketed to second place in the $2.2 billion OTC pain relief market, behind only Extra-Strength Tylenol.

Another drug that has racked up amazing profits by going OTC is the antihistamine Benadryl. In 1988 OTC Benadryl sales were $100 million, a fivefold increase over the drug's prescription-only sales of the year before.

The *Wall Street Journal* reported on June 5, 1988 that the mid nineties would experience the greatest number of changes ever from prescription to over-the-counter drugs. Jim Callandrill, a spokesman for Kline & Co., a New Jersey–based consulting firm, sees nonprescription drug sales soaring from $10 billion in 1988 to $38 billion in the next eleven years.

In part, this trend among the drug companies is simply an acknowledgment of marketing reality. Patent protection is set to expire in the next few years on many of the most widely used prescription drugs, exposing their makers to aggressive competition from manufacturers of generic drugs.

Under today's federal law, if a drug company is willing to finance and conduct the necessary testing to gain clearance on a drug for OTC status, that company can gain an extra three years exclusivity in marketing that drug, keeping the generics at bay long enough to establish brand-name loyalty. The success stories of Benadryl and Advil described above have been enough to convince most companies that accommodation is a wise course.

Even though many of the drugs scheduled to go OTC are stronger and carry greater risks of adverse side effects than prior OTC drugs, the die is cast. Over fifty current prescription drugs are now scheduled to reach OTC status in the next few years. These drugs include Zantac, Tagamet, Naprosyn, Seldane, Carafate, Pepcid, topical erythromycin, Nicorette, and 1 percent strength hydrocortisone.

If this change seems surprising, consider for a moment what is already happening in the rest of the world. Most other countries have very liberal regulations regarding which medications require prescription-only status. Only a few countries have the strict guidelines that exist in the United States, and these are largely northern European countries such as Great Britain and Scandinavia. But now even that is changing. For example, in 1989 Denmark moved fifty of its prescription drugs to OTC status.

Drug companies admit that today's medical consumer is more aware and conscious of health care issues than at any time in the past. "People are more educated about self-treatment possibilities," says Jean-Pierre Garnier, president of the US Pharmaceuticals division of Schering Plough Corporation of New Jersey.

According to the *Wall Street Journal*, Sidney Wolfe, who heads the Washington-based Health Research Group, agrees that consumers will benefit from giving OTC status to many prescription drugs: "On a case-by-case basis, if you can self-diagnose it makes sense to make these drugs available when appropriate . . . because these drugs are more effective than consumer treatments now available." In other words, most prescription drugs work better than current OTC remedies, so why not make them available at a reasonable price to those who need them?

THE NEW FDA RULING THAT
CAN MAKE A DIFFERENCE

Think of the pharmaceutical situation in the US as a vast network: the FDA, the American Medical Association, the local pharmacies, and the drug manufacturers all interacting to control the delivery of prescription drugs. For years this worked just fine. The United States had the most responsive system of health care in the world. Then came the explosion of health care costs—a complex and seemingly insoluble problem stemming from a variety of causes—along with the growing demand for treatment by groups of people suffering from rare diseases and the AIDS crisis, and everything suddenly fell apart.

All over the country people with AIDS began to openly defy the law. They didn't want to die while the drug companies and the FDA wasted time testing drugs that could potentially save their lives right now. And they complained about the unbelievably high costs of those drugs that were made available to them. AIDS victims began to go to other countries to get the drugs that they either couldn't get here or couldn't afford to buy. They even started their own clinical tests of promising new medications that they felt the FDA wasn't moving fast enough on.

Finally, the FDA had to admit what everyone else had known all along: the system simply wasn't working anymore. Today, more than ever before, those with the most urgent physical needs are getting the least. People have been either going without the treatments they need or foregoing other necessities in order to afford their medications.

And it's not only people suffering from AIDS who are unable to obtain or afford the drugs they need. Our own parents and grandparents are in the same boat. The need for effective, inexpensive medication has outgrown our mechanisms for developing and gaining approval for them.

The world of prescription drugs was never to be the same after FDA Commissioner Frank Young stepped up to the podium at the Tenth National Lesbian and Gay Health Conference and AIDS Forum in Boston, Massachusetts, on July 23, 1988. Young announced that from that point on, it would be perfectly legal for Americans to import *without a prescription* most foreign pharmaceuticals for personal use.

This FDA mail-import policy acknowledged what everyone had known for quite some time. And Young chose an audience that was ready, willing, and eager to hear about relief for their medical crisis. This group had been up in arms about the FDA's handling of the AIDS problem. The policy change meant that AIDS victims would no longer have to travel to Mexico, Japan, and other countries in order to legally obtain a treatment that might save or prolong their lives.

This FDA mail-import policy was formalized in the text of an FDA Talk Paper issued July 27, 1988, entitled "Policy on Importing Unapproved AIDS Drugs for Personal Use." It is reprinted here in its entirety.

On July 23, 1988, FDA Commissioner Frank E. Young, MD, PhD, addressed the Tenth National Lesbian and Gay Health Conference and AIDS Forum in Boston, Massachusetts, and answered questions. In his remarks he mentioned guidelines on the importation by mail of certain unapproved therapies outlined in a directive sent to FDA offices July 20, 1988, to clarify the status of those mail importations. The following may be used to answer questions:

For many years FDA has as a matter of discretion permitted individuals to bring into the US, for their personal use, quantities of drugs sold abroad but not approved in the US. Personal use quantities are generally considered to be amounts for a patient's treatment for three months or less. Imports involving larger quantities are generally not permitted as they lend themselves to commercialization.

Several unapproved drugs considered by some to be useful therapies for AIDS and AIDS-related conditions have been brought into the country by individual AIDS patients and their physicians for a number of years

23

under this policy. In most cases these products have been brought back through US Customs in the baggage of individuals returning from abroad.

Recently, however, some AIDS patients have attempted to mail or have mailed to them personal use quantities of dextran sulfate, a drug hoped to hold promise for treating AIDS, from Japan, where it has been marketed for years as a cholesterol-lowering agent. In order to assure that these mail shipments were handled in accordance with FDA importation policies, FDA's July 20 directive "Pilot Guidance for the Release of Mail Importation," sets forth, in the absence of unreasonable risk or fraud associated with a mailed product, the following conditions for permitting its importation:

- The product was purchased for personal use.
- The product is not for commercial distribution and the amount of product is not excessive (i.e., three-month supply or less).
- The intended use of the product is appropriately identified.
- The patient seeking to import the product affirms in writing that it is for the patient's own use and provides the name and address of the licensed physician in the US responsible for his or her treatment with the product.

This long-standing approach for releasing imported personal supplies has now been applied to most common medications, provided that they were not fraudulently promoted and did not present an unreasonable risk.

The July 20 guidance instructs FDA field offices to recommend that import alerts be issued for the automatic detention of imported products that do appear to be fraudulent or dangerous. Until an import alert is

24

issued, individuals importing will be informed in writing that the product may be detained unless it can be shown to meet the personal use entrance criteria as above.

FDA has forty import alerts advising both its field offices and the US Customs Service to restrict entry of medical products that are unsafe or clearly fraudulent. These alerts will continue to remain in effect and will continue to restrict the importation of such products as Laetrile, immuno-augmentative therapy agents, products promoted by Dr. Hans Nieper of West Germany, and products distributed by the Hauptmann Institute of Austria.

CURRENT FDA POLICY ON MEDICATION IMPORTATION

The document to which the above refers is reprinted in its entirety below, so that you can read for yourself the current FDA policy on importation of medications by mail.

July 20, 1988
FROM: Director, Office of Regional Operations
SUBJECT: Pilot Guidance for Release of Mail Importations
TO: Regional Food and Drug Directors, District Directors, Import Program Managers, Compliance Branch Managers, Investigations Branch Directors, Laboratory Branch Directors
INFO: All Major Field Offices, Resident Posts, Division of Field Science, Division of Federal-State Relations, Office of Legislative Affairs
NOTE: This guidance is being issued on a pilot

basis and is subject to change and/or cancellation. If the pilot proves successful, with no significant problems, Chapter 9-71 of the Regulatory Procedures Manual may be appropriately revised.

Because of the desire to acquire articles for treatment of serious and life-threatening conditions like AIDS and cancer, individuals have been purchasing unapproved products from foreign sources. Some of these products are sold over-the-counter in the country of origin, while others are available from clinics where the purchaser was treated. Such products are often shipped to the purchaser by mail.

Even though such products are subject to refusal, we may use our discretion to examine the background, risk, and purpose of these products before making a final decision. To assure that the districts are operating in a uniform manner, the following guidance is provided for dealing with personal use shipments.

1. Except as modified by these instructions, established guidance found in RPM-9-71, exhibits X9-71-1 and X9-71-2 should be followed.
2. A product entered for personal use, which meets the criteria in item 4 below, may proceed without sampling or detention.
3. Products that are not identified, or are not accompanied by documentation of intended use, should be detained. Other reasons for detention may include: size of the shipment (amount inconsistent with personal use), fraudulent promotion or misrepresentation, or an unreasonable health risk due to either toxicity or possible contamina-

tion. In such cases, the appropriate center should be contacted for guidance concerning release of the product.

4. Following detention, shipments may be released to an individual if the following criteria can be satisfied and there is no safety risk or evidence of fraud:
   a. The product was purchased for personal use.
   b. The product is not for commercial distribution and the amount of the drug is not excessive (i.e., a three-month supply or less).
   c. The intended use of the product is appropriately identified.
   d. The patient seeking to import the product affirms in writing that it is for the patient's own use and provides the name and address of the doctor licensed in the US responsible for his or her treatment with the product.

5. If the district should encounter a situation suggesting promotional and/or commercial activity that falls within our health fraud guideline, the district should recommend that an import alert be issued for the automatic detention of the product and identification of the promoter involved.

6. The model letter currently in exhibit X9-71-2 should be revised according to the attached during this pilot.

7. The article may then be *released with comment* upon receipt of the letter as follows:

MODEL LETTER FOR USE IN DRUG MAIL
EXHIBIT X9-71-2

A mail shipment of a drug from a foreign

country addressed to you is being detained at the post office. All products of this kind must meet the requirements of the Federal Food, Drug, and Cosmetic Act, which is designed to protect you from unsafe or misrepresented foods, drugs, cosmetics, and devices. Examination reveals that the product does not comply with the law.

Please read the enclosed Notice of Detention and Hearing carefully, since it explains why the product is believed to be in violation. The notice does not in any manner accuse you of violating any law.

If the drug is not approved for distribution in the US, it may be released for your personal use provided you furnish the following:

A letter providing adequate documentation that the product is for the patient's own use and the name and address of the doctor licensed in the United States responsible for his or her treatment with the product.

Send your statement to this office, and we will promptly review your submission and consider release of the product.

If you have good reason to believe the product does comply with the law and wish to discuss it with us, you may come personally to this office or write to us within the time limit shown on the notice.

If you do not wish to claim this shipment, you may disregard the notice and the shipment will be returned to sender without cost to you.

Sincerely yours,

Enclosure

WHAT DOES THIS NEW POLICY
MEAN FOR YOU?

Translated into everyday terms, the text of this mail import policy means that many of the most popular drugs such as Tagamet, minoxidil, Naprosyn, and common antibiotics such as amoxicillin, which require a prescription in the US, can now be ordered without a prescription from another country.

For the most part, Americans like you and me are now free to order, on our own, a personal, three-month supply of most popular drugs from any of a number of foreign sources, without sampling or detention by US Customs and without a doctor's prescription.

That also means that we are free to save big money. The standard medications that many of us are required to take over the course of our lifetime cost much less in other parts of the world. Foreign countries have lower drug costs because they don't carry the expensive overhead of the FDA approval process and physician controlled dispensing as in the US.

Further, you now have the freedom to order for your own use almost any drug on the market from foreign distributors. This decision is not just limited to AIDS medications; it applies to every drug in the world, as long as the drug is not a controlled substance (under DEA regulation) and is not considered harmful or fraudulent (under FDA alert restrictions). If, for example, you have a rare disease in which a drug used for its treatment has not been allowed on the market in the United States, you can now import the appropriate medications by mail order from other countries where they are available. The FDA mail import policy was greeted with joy in some circles, especially among the gay community, and with cynicism in others.

A 1988 article by Denise Grady and Doug M. Podolsky in *American Health* magazine reiterated that the new

FDA policy applied to *all* citizens, not only to those suffering from the AIDS virus. Now, people can import drugs of all descriptions to treat ailments ranging from cancer to arthritis. You can even import contraceptives by mail order.

The article emphasized that only the forty drugs already banned from the US by FDA import alert as dangerous or fraudulent are actually excluded from the new ruling. When the drug is intended for the personal use of the orderer, comprises only a three-month supply, and additionally, is taken under the guidance of a licensed US physician, the transaction is perfectly legal.

Of course the new policy has raised a lot of controversy among the medical and pharmaceutical establishments. It has caused many to speculate that the FDA itself, stunned by the consequences of the AIDS crisis, has simply thrown in the towel and abandoned its standards.

Newsweek, in its July 10, 1989 issue, trumpeted that after years of delays and unanswered pleas for faster drug approval, AIDS sufferers were at least able to gain an FDA response to their pleas for more timely access to new or foreign medications.

HOW CAN I USE THE NEW FDA RULING TO MY ADVANTAGE RIGHT NOW?

Quite simply, you can buy some of your medications, especially those which you take on a long-term basis, from international suppliers in other countries. It's not as convenient as going to your corner drugstore (if you are one of the few who has a corner drugstore anymore) but it can be almost as fast with modern technologies such as international telephone, fax service, credit cards that are accepted worldwide, and overnight air express service.

The big cost savings that this approach can bring may be worth the extra wait. Plus you don't have to visit your doctor to get refills of your prescription each time that you order.

As anyone who has traveled to Europe, Mexico, South America, or the Far East has already discovered, other countries in the world dispense a broad range of popular medications directly from the pharmacy to the consumer without the high cost or the long delays that are involved with a visit to the doctor.

Around the world, such well-known pharmaceuticals as Tagamet, Zantac, and Flagyl are commonly sold over the counter in local pharmacies. From birth control pills to antibiotics, most medications are available without prescription. Consumers save tremendously on their overall health bills because they don't pay for excessive visits to doctors.

For example, in the United States, hydrocortisone at 1 percent concentration, requires a doctor's prescription. In almost every other country in the world, it is an OTC drug and always has been. Here, the only way to obtain a prescription for 1 percent hydrocortisone is to visit your doctor, at a cost of about $65 per visit, and then pay your pharmacist another $10 to $15 for a little tube of cream. That's not to mention the lost work time, travel to and from the doctor's office, and time spent in the waiting room. Thus, getting the medication to clear up a simple skin irritation may cost an American upwards of $100.

A British, French, or Greek person with the same skin condition pays about $2.50 to his local pharmacist for the same medicine, often produced by an international branch of the same drug company. That is a savings of over 90 percent from what we pay in America. No wonder the United States spends so much of its gross national product on health care!

But what about safety? That is the concern of most individuals when they first hear this information. If people are allowed to get their medications directly from the pharmacist, instead of spending $65 for a trip to the doctor's office to get a prescription, isn't there a big medical risk involved? Absolutely not. In other countries, with these more liberal prescription policies, life expectancy figures are similar to and even better than those found in the US.

And experience with this kind of system has been positive enough that even more countries are now moving to liberalize prescription laws rather than to tighten them. The only ones to complain have been a few members of the medical community who are either extremely conservative or who fear possible loss of income.

CHAPTER II

How Can I Purchase Medications from Other Countries?

At this point in the book you might be asking, "How and where do I place my order?" That's what this book is all about. In Appendix I you will find a listing of pharmaceutical companies (including addresses and phone numbers) that are willing to sell personal quantities of medications via mail order.

Please note that none of these pharmaceutical companies advertise to the American public. Most were even reluctant to have me print anything about their services. Their reasoning is straightforward. According to the FDA ruling you can buy drugs by mail from sources outside the United States only if you were not solicited by that source. The rationale for this twist in the ruling isn't clear to me, and it seems very convoluted, but it is a fact.

The organizations listed in this book are greatly concerned that they comply with all FDA regulations. They live in fear that their shipments filling orders for drugs to the United States can be detained by an FDA action against them. So don't expect these places to send you a catalog. They can fill your orders, but that is all they can do.

I sent out more than 2000 questionnaires worldwide to locate the few companies who were willing to take a chance on being listed in this book. In all cases I found these sources by referral and got them to agree to be listed by begging and cajoling. I argued that they could have faith in the American system of fairness. I told them that the US Constitution guards against ex post facto legislation.

I am not in a position to recommend any of these companies. Their names and addresses are presented for informational purposes only. I have personally tried all of them and had no difficulties. In fact, their service has been very good. The medications that they sent have worked like any others I have taken. However, the same results may not occur for you.

Wherever possible, I've included ordering instructions and prices in US dollars as well. These prices are accurate as of June 30, 1990. Expect them to change over time. Things always do! So call or write to verify before you order. Here's how you can place an order with one of these firms or any others that you might learn about.

First, you must make up your own order form. Remember, it is *illegal* for foreign pharmaceutical firms to solicit you in any way. So you should make up your own form or copy the one that is presented on the next page. (I have used this one everywhere and it works fine. Also, it complies with all aspects of the FDA's import guidelines.) Ask that the pharmacy include a copy of your order with the return shipment to avoid any problems with US Customs.

Mail Purchase Order for Importing Pharmaceuticals as Allowed under FDA "Pilot Guidance" Dated July 20, 1988

Name _____

Address _____

City _____ State _____ ZIP _____

Telephone Number _____ Fax Number _____

Drug Name   Intended Use   Quantity   Price

_____

_____

_____

Shipping Instructions _____

_____

Shipping Charges _____

Total _____

Amount of Money Order Enclosed _____

Name of Supervising Physician _____

I certify that I am ordering these drugs for personal use only for a period of less than ninety days.

Signature _____

Please bill my MasterCard# _____

VISA# _____ American Express# _____

Expiration Date _____

CHAPTER III

Buying Pharmaceuticals Directly in Mexico and the Caribbean

GETTING STARTED IN MEXICO

The text of the new FDA ruling makes clear that you can bring back personal quantities of most drugs as part of your luggage if you travel to a foreign country. All you need do is declare this fact to customs officials on your return to the United States. For some people this will probably be the preferred way to take advantage of the FDA's money-saving ruling.

If you are like many Americans, you can more than pay for a trip to Mexico with the savings that you will make on a personal three-month supply of regular prescription medications. Mexico has some of the best pharmaceutical prices in the world.

Take my own case for example. Through my physician I have regular prescriptions for Tenormin and Dyazide for hypertension, Mevocor for high cholesterol, and Tagamet for ulcers. The cost of a three-month supply at my local drugstore in northern California is $325. The cost for these same medications in Tijuana is just $135. That means I can save $190 just by shopping in Mexico.

Even if I include air fare to San Diego, a trolley trip to the border, taxi fares, and food, my total expenses for a day trip are less than $100. That means an actual out-of-pocket savings of about $90 every three months for my standard ongoing prescriptions. Plus, I get the fun of a day's outing that is paid for by my savings.

But what about the quality? The generally prevailing view is probably that of Gordon McGuire, head pharmacist of the University of California at San Diego Medical Center. In an article that appeared in the *San Diego Union* on November 11, 1986, McGuire expressed the view that quality control was not as effective in Mexico as it was in the US and that in fact many people had entered the San Diego Medical Center suffering from reactions or symptoms that could be related to medications they had obtained in Mexico.

I hate to be a heretic, but it is hard for me to accept this kind of thinking. There are several reasons why I can't go along with it. First, I disagree on logical grounds. If people are going to get sick from Mexican medications, why doesn't it happen to the citizens of Mexico themselves? It is logically impossible for me to believe that there is a whole medical-pharmaceutical complex in Mexico that has a mission of making people sick rather than healthy.

Second, if it is true, then you would think that the death rate in Mexico should be a lot higher than it is in the United States. But actually just the opposite is true. According to the United Nations, Monthly Health Statistics, May 1989, the crude yearly death rate figures per 1000 population during 1980 were 6.2 for Mexico and 8.9 for the United States.

Finally, I have bought and used Mexican pharmaceuticals on numerous occasions and have never had any side effects. (I know this is not a strong argument by itself, but let me go on.) These medications are from major drug companies such as Smith Kline & French, Parke-Davis, CIBA/GEIGY, and Glaxo. I don't mean to say that a brand name is all that important, just that these products look just like what I buy in the States. And, in fact, they work just like the ones that I get in the States.

I suspect what lies behind such fears is a lurking prejudice against Mexican cleanliness. The question probably goes like this, "How do you expect me to trust the pharmaceuticals made in a country where you can get dysentery from drinking the water?" That is a good question. And it is up to each individual to decide that for himself. All I can say is that it doesn't bother me. I personally have never had a problem nor met another American who has had a problem, but then who am I to say? If the UC San Diego Medical School Center is overrun with such cases, I must be wrong. That is, if it is overrun with such cases.

If you decide for yourself that Mexican-produced drugs are all right and you want to save money, then go to Mexico and test the system. In all likelihood you will go to one of the border towns such as Tijuana (from San Diego), Nogales (from Tucson), Juarez (from El Paso), or Laredo (from San Antonio) to make your purchases. Another good alternative is to take a nice beach vacation to Acapulco, Cancun, Mazatlan, Puerto Vallarta, or one of the other wonderful resort areas in Mexico.

While most Mexican and US officials deny it, many, many people cross the border on a regular basis to save money on the purchase of their regular medications. Just take a look at a quote from a popular tourist guide for Tijuana, Mexico:

Hundreds of Americans travel across the border every week to buy drugs—legally. In the US the same items would require a prescription. Some drugs would be unobtainable in the US except for controlled experiments, because the US Food and Drug Administration has not approved them for sale yet. But in Tijuana, as well as in the rest of Mexico and in some other countries, they are readily available. The reason is that in countries which have lower standards of living, it is believed better for the sufferer to be able to buy the drug than to pass it up because he can't afford to visit a doctor. In the long run, they feel this benefit out-

39

weighs the risk of obtaining the wrong drug. In Mexico, a druggist himself will recommend the proper drug to buy, or he can (and will) refuse a drug he thinks you shouldn't have. Drugs for sale include everything from birth control pills (the birth control pill was invented in Mexico) to pain killers, antidepressants, antiarthritics, diet pills, heart medications, etc. You can get drugs for AIDS ailments, steroids, hormones, drugs for psychotic disorders, antidiuretics, muscle relaxants, and even simple cold remedies. (p. 234, *Having Fun in Tijuana* by Sam Warren.)

It is evident to anyone who crosses the border into Mexico that there are scores of pharmacies that are loaded with boxes, tubes, and jars of medications that are sold on a prescription-only basis in the United States. And all types of people, including many Americans, are walking into these pharmacies and buying these pharmaceuticals without prescriptions. I've seen it done over and over.

In many cases you will find that there is not a pharmacist on the premises. Mexican law allows pharmacists to oversee as many as three pharmacies. So for the most part expect to buy your medications from shop clerks who have received all their training on the job.

Therefore, only a rare individual will want to experiment with new medications. Most people will opt for the prudent route and only purchase those drugs already prescribed by their US physician. If you take a conservative approach, my experience is that you will be perfectly safe and you will save a lot of money.

I have purchased drugs that are prescription only in the US on an OTC basis on numerous occasions in Tijuana, Juarez, Puerto Vallarta, Mazatlan, and Acapulco. Never once have I had any kind of problem in buying pharmaceuticals without a prescription or a problem with the quality of the drugs dispensed.

Of these four locations, I much prefer Tijuana. There

are three times as many pharmacies in Tijuana as there are in Mazatlan, Puerto Vallarta, Juarez, and Acapulco together. The pharmacies there are bigger, better stocked, and more likely to have English-speaking personnel. Some even have pharmacists on hand, and clearly they want to sell to Americans.

Despite the fact that Juarez has a population greater than one million, it has relatively few drugstores by Tijuana standards. Those that you do find tend to be small, understocked, and staffed by people who only speak Spanish. But, still, druggists in Juarez are extremely helpful. For example, in one case a druggist sent a runner to fetch a bottle of one hundred Tagamet tablets for me because he only had forty tablets left in stock.

Acapulco and Mazatlan are my least favorite Mexican stops for pharmaceutical buying. They are great for vacationing, but their selection of drugstores is very poor and oriented toward tourist-related illness. These medications, however, are easily available everywhere. For example, the gift shop at the Princess Hotel in Acapulco carries Lomotil.

BUYING PHARMACEUTICALS IN THE CARIBBEAN

When you walk into the average drugstore in the Caribbean you are surprised at how much it looks like an American pharmacy. There is generally an OTC section and then a prescription area that is somewhat raised above the rest of the floor with a glassed-in counter. Usually there is a man dressed in a starched white uniform who stands behind the counter. Often he is a US-trained pharmacist.

Until recently, I was sure that these pharmacies operated exactly the way that they do in the United States. I thought medicines were dispensed by prescription only.

But I was shaken from this belief while reading two of the FDA's many import alerts.

The first alert to catch my eye was dated September 17, 1982. It concerned a ban on the import of the antiaging product called Gerovital. The alert said that people were importing Gerovital from Grand Cayman Island in the British West Indies. The second alert was dated July 14, 1988 and concerned the banning of the import of immunoaugmentive drugs from Freeport in the Bahamas.

It seemed to me that if these countries allowed drugstores to mail these controversial drugs to the United States without prescriptions, then they were likely to have very liberal pharmaceutical laws about the need for a medical prescription if you walked into a pharmacy.

Given that the Caribbean islands are most frequent travel destinations for Americans living in the East, Southeast, and Midwest than is Mexico, I decided to visit Freeport in the Bahamas and Grand Cayman Island to see for myself how their drugstores operated.

The result was a pleasant trip to Freeport and Grand Cayman. My first observation about the pharmacies in both of these countries was that they didn't look at all like those in Mexico. Just as I remembered, they are like the ones here in the United States.

On both islands the responses from all druggists that I checked were the same. First, the pharmacist asked for a prescription. When I replied that I didn't have one because I was on vacation, they were glad to provide what I asked for.

I talked to these pharmacists about their prices. They said that they pay much less for their pharmaceuticals than drugstores pay in the States and they claimed that their prices are much lower. They indicated that they would be very happy to help me save money by selling ninety-day quantities.

However, it looks to me like Caribbean prices are higher than Mexico's and sometimes even higher than the prices in the US. So if you plan on saving money by buying pharmaceuticals in the Caribbean, you should first price shop at home and then comparison shop while you are vacationing. Whether or not you will save money by shopping for your medications in the islands appears to be very hit and miss.

All in all, the Caribbean just doesn't have the positive feel that you get when you are in Tijuana. (Of course, that is also true of the Mexican resorts.) The drugstores are not well stocked, and you don't feel as if you are getting a bargain.

Sorting it all out, then, my own personal view is as follows. If you decide to travel to one of the United States' southern neighbors to save money on your medications, Tijuana is still your best bet. It has good prices and good services.

Just remember, before deciding to go, that many experts have grave concerns about the quality of Mexican pharmaceuticals. So think carefully. There may be risk involved.

CHAPTER IV

What If I Am Less Concerned about Costs and More Concerned about Getting Treatment for a Rare Disorder?

Congress enacted the Orphan Drug Act in 1983 and amended it in 1984. What the act did was address that situation in which people with rare diseases are not able to acquire medicine to treat their condition.

An "orphan" disease is defined as one that affects 200,000 or less people. There are approximately twenty-one "orphan disease" advocacy groups who helped bring about the passage of the Orphan Drug Act, organizations representing people with such conditions as Lou Gehrig's disease, Gilles de la Tourette's syndrome, Wilson's disease, myoclonus and many genetically transmitted diseases.

Because these rare diseases affect only a comparatively small number of people, pharmaceutical companies have seldom found it possible to go through the traditional FDA approval process to develop new treatments and make money in the process.

This has led to our definition of "orphan" drugs. An orphan drug is any drug that has been developed abroad and is commercially available overseas, but which is not being marketed by a US company. An orphan drug may also be a natural substance that cannot be patented by law and which pharmaceutical companies are therefore not interested in.

When the Orphan Drug Act was passed, its provisions made it possible for the government, through grants and tax incentives, to underwrite the development of drugs for rare diseases. The financial value of these substances to the company might be small, but their humanitarian value is great.

The act also paves the way for acceptance of overseas clinical research data on drugs, so that all foreign testing does not have to be repeated in the United States in order to meet FDA guidelines.

The Orphan Drug Act set up the Office of Orphan Drug Development. This agency is supposed to oversee the introduction of the new drugs and the carrying out of the limited number of tests that were now required to get new drugs to the people who need them.

However, there are many who feel that the Orphan Drug Act has not fulfilled its intention of making new, rare, or foreign drugs more easily available for use by the people who need them. From 1983 through 1987, the Office of Orphan Drugs had approved only thirteen drugs for marketing out of one hundred requests filed.

An interesting coincidence is that during this same time, congress also passed a bill making it legal for pharmaceutical companies to market drugs abroad if they have not received FDA approval in the United States. The message this sends is that even though the pharmaceutical companies consider these drugs effective enough to be sold abroad, US citizens cannot use them legally.

One of the reasons for the slow pace of US approval of new orphan drugs is the difficulty that manufacturers have in gaining insurance protection for the introduction of new drugs. Another reason is that there still exists a very high cost to a pharmaceutical company that wishes to begin testing the effectiveness of a new drug from overseas. This cost, more than $125,000, effectively eliminates most small companies from developing and marketing orphan drugs.

HOW DO I OBTAIN MEDICATIONS THAT HAVE NOT YET BEEN APPROVED ACCORDING TO THE ORPHAN DRUG ACT?

Now that the FDA allows you to import drugs from other countries, there is finally a solution to this problem. It is about the only way in which many people in the United States with very rare diseases will ever obtain an appropriate treatment. The only other choice is to pick up and move to a country that has an effective treatment on the market.

Chapter IX is a compilation of some orphan drugs, not yet available in the United States, that I think are particularly interesting. Keep in mind that there are many more such drugs that are alternative therapies for other rare medical conditions. People with orphan diseases should, of course, seek treatment under the guidance of their own physicians. This listing includes the action of the drug, usual dosage, and side effects.

For more complete information on this subject I strongly recommend that you get a copy of *Orphan Drugs: Your Complete Guide to Effective Tested Medications Outside the US—and Their Availability* by Kenneth and Lois Anderson. It is published by the Body Press, a division of Price Stern Sloan, 360 North La Cienega Boulevard, Los Angeles, CA 90048. This book lists nearly two hundred drugs that have passed scientific study in other countries, but not in the US. It also gives the names and addresses of two hundred forty-one foreign pharmaceutical manufacturers who sell these drugs.

However, you should be aware that most of these big international manufacturers will not fill orders on an individual basis. Fortunately, there is a very helpful pharmaceutical distributor in Tijuana, Mexico, who you can call for help:

Bomuca SA de CV
Avenue De Los Pollos 26-C
La Mesa, Tijuana, B.C. Mexico 22456

Their phone number is 52-66-216074, and it can be direct dialed from anywhere in the United States. The staff speaks excellent English. If they carry the product you need, they can send it via overnight air mail.

If they don't carry the product that you need, ask to speak to their director general. He has contacts with international pharmaceutical distributors around the world, so he can probably order what you need. This organization got started by delivering AIDS medications to physicians in the United States. It has many regular customers who are physicians.

In addition to Bomuca, I have learned recently of another distributor who is extremely helpful and willing to ship to the United States. This company maintains an order-taking answering service and mail pickup just north of the Mexican border, so it is especially convenient to order from them. Their service is fast and they accept checks. Their specialty seems to be memory enhancers, treatments for colds and flu, and unusual treatments for cancer and other serious diseases. If you write or call, they will send a listing of their products:

Pharmaceuticals International
539 Telegraph Canyon Road, Suite 227
Chula Vista, CA 92010-6436
Telephone: 1-800-365-3698

CHAPTER V

What about the Drugs that I Cannot Order by Mail?

CONTROLLED SUBSTANCES

You cannot purchase what the DEA terms "controlled substances" by mail without a physician's prescription. And some controlled substances, such as schedule I drugs listed below, are not allowed into the country *with or without* a physician's prescription.

Controlled substances fall under the jurisdiction of the DEA (Drug Enforcement Administration) which works jointly with the FDA to regulate drugs coming into the US. Controlled substances are listed under several classifications, called *schedules*.

These schedules came about as a result of a law called the Comprehensive Drug Abuse Prevention and Control Act of 1970. But the actual history of antinarcotics legislation reaches much farther back than that. The growth of this body of law runs parallel to the FDA legislation and often overlaps it.

Let's take a broad overview of drugs in the US and see how the laws and schedules came into existence.

Schedule I

Drugs that are schedule I have a high potential for abuse and have *no* currently acceptable medical use in the United States. Such drugs include heroin, marijuana, peyote, mescaline, psilocybin, tetrahydrocannabinols, LSD, ketobemidone, levomoramide, racemoramide, benzylmorphine, dihydromorphine, morphine methylsulfonate, nicocodeine, nicomorphine, methaqualone, and others. These substances are sometimes obtained for research and instructional use if medical personnel apply to the Drug Enforcement Administration. It is *always* illegal to possess these drugs, and you may not order them under any circumstances or receive them in the mail.

Schedule II

Schedule II drugs have a high abuse potential, with an extreme danger of causing psychic or physical dependence. Schedule II controlled substances consist of certain opiates, and drugs containing methamphetamine as the single active ingredient or in combination with other drugs. Examples of such drugs are opium, morphine, codeine, hydromorphone, methadone, meperidine, cocaine, oxycodone, anileridine, oxymorphone, dextroamphetamine, and methamphetamine. Also included are phenmetrazine, methylphenidate, amobarbital, pentobarbital, secobarbital, etorphine hydrochloride, and diphenoxylate.

Schedule III

The drugs in this schedule are less addictive than those above, but also have a high potential for abuse and dependence, leading to moderate or low physical addiction but a high degree of psychological addiction. This schedule includes compounds containing limited quantities of certain opiates and even nonopiate drugs such as chlorhexadol, glutethimide, methyprylon, sulfondiethylmethane, sulfonmethan, nalorphine, benzphetamine, chlorphentermine, chlortermine, phendimetrazine, and certain barbiturates not listed in other schedules.

Schedule IV

The drugs on this schedule actually have a low potential for abuse that can lead to limited physical dependence or psychological dependence. These drugs include barbital, phenobarbital, methylphenobarbital, chloral betain, chloral hydrate, ethchlorvynol, ethinamate, meprobamate, paraldehyde, methohexital, fenfluramine, diethylpropion, phentermine, the benzodiazepines, mebutamate, and propoxyphene.

Schedule V

The drugs in schedule V have a lesser potential for abuse than those in schedule IV and generally are composed of lower proportions of opiates or psychoactive elements than those above. These preparations may be for coughs, colds, or diarrhea, and may be dispensed without a prescription provided that such distribution is made by a registered pharmacist and include not more than 24 milliliters of any schedule V substance containing opium, nor more than 120 milliliters or more than twenty-four solid dosage units of any other controlled substance that is sold to the same customer in any given forty-eight-hour period without a valid prescription order; a record book is maintained that contains the name and address of the purchaser, name and quantity of the controlled substance sold, date of sale, and the initials of the pharmacist.

Packages must display the following words: "Caution: Federal law prohibits the transfer of this drug to any person other than the patient for whom it was prescribed." Section 1311.27 of the federal drug law describes the only exemptions made for personal use of DEA controlled drugs as follows:

Any individual who has in his possession a controlled substance listed in schedules II, III, IV, or V, which he has lawfully obtained for his personal medical use, or for administration to an animal accompanying him, may enter or depart the United States with such substance notwithstanding sections 1002-1005 of the Act (21 USC 952-955), providing the following conditions are met:

a. the controlled substance is in the original container in which it was dispensed to the individual

b. the individual makes a declaration to an appropriate official of the US Customs Service stating:

c. that the controlled substance is possessed for his personal use or for an animal accompanying him

d. the trade or chemical name and the symbol designating the schedule of the controlled substance if it appears on the container label, or, if such names do not appear on the label, the name and address of the pharmacy or practitioner who dispensed the substance, and the prescription number, if any.

Whether or not these same exemptions apply to mail-order importation is still unclear. Some officials that I talked to at the FDA thought that they did. But everyone that I talked to at the DEA disagreed. Given that there are serious criminal penalties (like a year or more in jail) for the illegal importation of DEA controlled substances, it is better to take the most conservative approach possible. Therefore, I am not including any information about these medications in this volume.

Obviously, the intent of the law is not to prevent people who actually need a medicine from bringing in a personal supply; it is only to prevent people from importing huge quantities and selling them illegally. The new FDA ruling only expands this philosophy. You may import by mail order a *personal*, or three-month supply of your medication without bringing upon yourself legal consequences.

The Narcotic Drugs—Uses and Abuses

If you're curious why these drugs among all others, provoke such a powerful sanction, let's look at the nature and history of a few narcotics. Since the beginning of recorded time, and no doubt before that, every society has used drugs in some form or another with the intention of producing an alteration in state of mind or body. Whether these substances are alcohol, opiates, psychedelics, amphetamines, or other, milder ones, this always seems to have been the case. The use of drugs for nonmedical purposes is as old as civilization.

Why Do People Take Narcotic Drugs?

Drugs serve a variety of purposes, both legal and non-legal, approved and disapproved. They relieve pain; tranquilize the mind, bring about sleep; relieve coughing; and give a feeling of well-being, euphoria, or relief from anxiety. Narcotics can also produce many side effects, such as constipation, anxiety, restlessness, fear, nausea, vomiting, dizziness, and shortness of breath. Overdoses cause depression of the nervous and respiratory system, coma, and death.

All narcotics are addicting. People who regularly take one of these drugs will experience the phenomenon of addiction, including tolerance to the drug (requiring larger doses to achieve the same effect) and withdrawal symptoms such as trembling, nausea, sweating, hallucinations, anxiety, and sometimes seizures when the drug is removed.

Since the definition of drug abuse is a cultural and social one, there is naturally a large variation among societies and cultures as to what constitutes a drug problem. For example, a mild degree of alcohol intoxication is acceptable in Western cultures, but is forbidden in the Middle Eastern Moslem culture.

Besides medical drug use, nonmedical drug use may consist of social, experimental, or circumstantial drug use. It is when the use of the drug becomes compulsive or out of the control of the individual that we call the behavior drug-addicted.

53

One of the hazards in using drugs is that the nature of the substance and the feeling it produces can promote dependency. The intensity of this dependency may vary from mild to desperate. One thing is certain: the addict experiences changes in body and mind that give the feeling that being without the drug is unendurable. Thus, the addict is willing to exert every effort possible to acquire the drug, even at great personal risk and endangerment of others.

What Makes Narcotic Drugs Act as They Do?

The most frequently used narcotics have been opium, morphine, heroin, and codeine. But there are also many synthetic or nonopiate narcotics.

Raw opium is a natural product. It consists of the juice of the unripe capsule of the opium poppy. The chief active ingredient in opium is morphine. Heroin is produced by the chemical reaction that takes place when morphine is heated with acetic acid, a chemical found in common vinegar. The body rapidly converts the heroin back into morphine. The drug codeine is also present in opium in small amounts. Examples of synthetic, or manufactured, opiates are methadone and meperidine.

There are many different ways that these drugs can find their way into the body. They can be taken orally, smoked, sniffed, or injected under the skin or into a vein or muscle. Narcotics act primarily on the central nervous system, but they may affect many other organs and systems. The liabilities of drug addiction are both physiological and social.

DRUGS ON THE FDA IMPORT ALERT LISTS

Besides the DEA-controlled substances, the FDA also issues documents called *import alerts*. You cannot legally import any drug which is on the import alert list.

Drugs banned from import by the FDA include: tuberculosis vaccine from Japan that is thought to cure cancer, herpes virus vaccine, all drugs from the Hauptmann Institute in Austria, cellular therapies such as those developed by Neihans in Switzerland, chloramphenicol, Gerovital, immunoaugmentative therapy for cancer developed by Dr. Burton, Diennet Diet Pills, germanium based drugs, Laetrile, methapyrilene, anabolic steroids of any kind, Tagamet from Canada, human plasma and serum, interferon, vitamin B-15, DMSO, many crude drugs from China, Oil of Evening Primrose, homeopathic cancer drugs by Erich Klemko, adrenal cortex extract, Woodward's Gripe Water, green lipped mussel as a treatment for arthritis, Eagle Medicated Oil, Padma 28, starch blockers, *azoque* and similar Mexican folk medicines, Tatex tattoo remover, P2P, Catha Edulis, Matol, CU-7 Intrauterine Contraceptive Device, Rivixil, Comycin, Redotex Diet Pills, danthron, antiaging creams, THA, clozapine, and RU 486.

For the most part, these are drugs that are fraudulent, dangerous, or have not been tested enough to determine their effectiveness. It is thought that they may pose direct or indirect health hazards. In some cases, as I mentioned earlier, import alerts are purely political.

The total list of import alerts includes medications of all kinds, as well as certain foodstuffs from abroad that may contain insect pests, poisons such as mercury, funguses, or other dangers to the American public or environment. Misleadingly labelled products are also kept out.

The process of creating an import alert is actually a very ad hoc event. A large number of people within the FDA have the authority to start an investigation that could lead to the issuance of an alert. In fact, it appears that anyone on the FDA staff can get the ball rolling. And, even more surprisingly, quite a number of people within the FDA can approve an alert as a legal United States government ruling.

In most cases the import alert process is neither overseen nor even signed off by the FDA commissioner. One high ranking official in the FDA told me that the last import alert he remembered the commissioner approving was one that had to do with foods from China. There was concern that there could be large political repercussions with the Chinese government because such an alert could greatly damage the economy of a small section of China.

Some alerts are obviously the result of a call from a big drug manufacturer to people inside the agency. (An example of this is the ban on the importation of Tagamet from Canada on the "grounds" of safety!) Others probably resulted from political or religious pressure.

Be sure to check with the FDA yourself from time to time if you want to make sure of the mail import policy. There is no way to guess when an import alert is going to appear next. So to be safe, call the FDA to make sure that they have not decided to ban one of the medications you might wish to import by mail.

I have included an abridged version of all the relevant import alerts in Appendix II because it is almost impossible to get a copy from the FDA. The first few times I asked, I was told that I would have to file for a copy under the Freedom of Information Act. The people who I talked to said that there are no copies to send out to ordinary citizens.

I managed to get one straight thinking member of the FDA to make copies of the alerts for me on his own time. Thanks to this official you can know specifically what is banned from import by FDA alert.

Read Appendix II carefully if you are thinking about importing any of the drugs that are not listed in the next four chapters. The drugs listed in this book are approved by the FDA or the DEA for mail-order importation. But remember, when in doubt, it is always wise to call the FDA first.

CHAPTER VI

Some Things You Should Understand about Taking Any Medication

A drug is something you put in your body that is going to affect or alter the way your body functions. There is no such thing as a drug that has *no effect*. Even though you may not be aware of everything that is taking place inside your body, the drug you have taken will influence your body functions in some way. That is why it is especially important to understand your condition and to be sure that you take the proper drug in the proper amount for the condition that you have. Remember that each person is a unique individual with a body chemistry that is like nobody else's. Any drug you take will be reacting on you and you alone.

The best way to ensure that you are taking a drug properly is to consult your physician and your pharmacist. These people are highly trained health professionals, who are the most reliable source of up-to-date information on your condition and the drug that is appropriate to treat it.

DRUG ALLERGIES

If you have once been allergic to a drug, you may be sure that you will always be allergic to it. Allergies do not change with age or go away if you do not use a drug for a period of time. Allergic reactions can range all the way from a mild rash to anaphylaxis—a literal shutdown of your body processes that can be life threatening if not treated at once.

Always let your physician know if you have shown an allergic reaction to a drug in the past. Never experiment with a drug that you suspect you may be allergic to. Often being allergic to one drug can make you allergic to that whole family of drugs and to related drug families as well. If you have reacted allergically to one form of penicillin, you should not take any form of penicillin, and you also may be allergic to a family of drugs called the cephalosporins. Be sure to consult with your doctor before taking any medication.

SENSITIVITY AND SIDE EFFECTS ARE DIFFERENT THAN ALLERGIES

Side effects are unexpected or unwanted reactions of your body to a certain drug. Drowsiness, for example, is a side effect of many drugs used to treat allergies. Side effects may be a minor inconvenience or may be so severe that you will want to switch to another form of medication. Most side effects are minor, compared to the benefits you gain from the drug, but you will want to stay in close touch with your doctor and follow his or her advice regarding driving, operating machinery, or performing other tasks that may require alertness.

Here are some important things to remember about side effects when you are taking drugs.

Your age influences the action of the drugs you take. Children under twelve years old will respond differently to drugs than someone who is older. And children under two years old respond significantly different to drugs in most cases. Not only your age, but your sex and physical condition make you more or less sensitive to various drugs. For example, people over seventy years old may be more sensitive to the effects of tranquilizers than adolescents. These older people tend to experience more side effects from their medication in general. For this reason as well, you should be in close contact with the prescribing doctor at all times during the course of your medication and immediately report any unusual reactions.

Elderly people are especially vulnerable to being overmedicated. If you are a senior, you should be aware yourself of the normal processes of aging; that the liver and kidneys may metabolize some drugs differently, causing toxic effects from what would be a moderate dosage in someone younger. Aspirin, for example, may be retained in greater quantities by the elderly because it is not excreted by the kidneys as efficiently as in younger people. Aspirin overdose can cause confusion, ringing in the ears, deafness, and irritability. Make sure your physician is knowledgeable about the special needs of geriatric patients and the practice of wise geriatric medicine.

If you are taking more than one drug, the drugs may interact with one another. Drug interactions may take several forms. They may make one another stronger, or weaken and cancel one another's effects. Drug interactions do this often by slowing the body's rate of absorption of drugs taken at the same time. Some drugs will stimulate the faster release of other drugs in the body. Drugs that are broken down in the liver will often do this. The drug's action can be affected, causing a potential overdose reaction even though you have taken the prescribed amount.

Sometimes one drug will cause another drug to be eliminated from the body more rapidly. Since many drugs are eliminated by the kidneys, the condition of a person's kidneys obviously affects the time of elimination and the amount that can be processed and excreted.

Some drugs will react against one another, simply by their very nature. Antidepressants and sedatives, for example, will "fight" with one another. You must be very careful to understand the action of the drugs you take. It is often a wise idea to consult both your doctor and your pharmacist in order to be sure you understand all of the potential reactions to your medications. In this book we have tried to list common drug interactions, but this is a large and complex topic. Your doctor and pharmacist are still the best sources for current information about drug interactions.

INTERACTIONS THAT HEIGHTEN THE EFFECT OF A DRUG

A drug interaction that increases the effect of another drug is called potentiation. There are many chemical processes that take place in the body that may work to accomplish this. Some drugs cause other drugs to be released faster. Because of this, your dose of the first drug may need to be cut if you begin taking the second. Some antidiabetes drugs react this way with sulfa drugs. They can cause a drop of blood sugar by working too well since there is actually too much of the drug in your system at one time. Your doctor will probably adjust your medication.

Again, the condition of a person's kidneys will affect how rapidly a drug is excreted. Also, some drugs affect the kidneys to interfere with the processing of other drugs. For example, the drug probenecid interferes with the elimination of penicillin by the kidneys and causes a rise in the amount of penicillin in the bloodstream.

The most common of drug interactions is of one drug with the same drug. This is called an additive effect. In other words, if you take more of a certain drug, or take another dose before the action of the first has completely been eliminated, you will experience a higher level of effect, and some reactions or side effects of that drug that occur usually at higher doses may set in. It is critical that you take your medication according to the schedule prescribed by your doctor. Do not try to judge whether a drug is still working by how you feel, as the drug may still be present in your bloodstream and taking more could result in an overdose. Always consult your doctor if you feel you are not receiving the full benefits of your medication.

Elderly people who may be taking a large number of drugs are particularly at risk for drug interactions. Even such seemingly nonreactive substances as vitamin pills may cause a difference in the way your body reacts to a certain medication. It seems that as we age, our bodies are quicker to respond to most drugs, and this sets up an environment for adverse reactions.

Many foods can cause a drug to be absorbed or processed differently by your body. Some drugs must be taken on an empty stomach in order to have their greatest effect; others must be taken on a full stomach to prevent irritation. Food generally prolongs the time it takes for a drug to get into your bloodstream. This is because most drugs are absorbed through the wall of the stomach or the intestine, and food naturally interferes with the drug reaching that area. However, eventually the drug will probably be absorbed, so food does not prevent the action of the drug entirely. While taking drugs on a full stomach may be necessary sometimes to prevent irritation, you will probably take most drugs on an empty stomach.

Some foods will interfere with the absorption of drugs. This is why people are told not to take milk with tetracycline, but to wait several hours. Sometimes vitamins or foods containing a high amount of a certain vitamin will affect the action of a drug. Therefore, while taking some drugs, such as anticoagulants, you will probably be advised to cut your consumption of green, leafy vegetables which contain high amounts of vitamin K, the vitamin that helps blood to clot. Be sure to follow your doctor's instructions as to diet when taking any and all medications.

You may have or develop an allergy to a drug, even if you have taken it safely before. You must always be alert to any abnormal or unexpected reactions that occur after you have taken a drug. There is a difference between a side effect of a drug and an allergic reaction to that drug. A side effect may make a drug intolerable and necessitate a change of prescription, but that is still different from an allergic reaction, which may need medical treatment.

Whenever you add a drug or change your medication, your doctor or pharmacist should reassess all of the medications you are taking in order to make sure that some new potential interactions will not take place or will be minimized. Sometimes the dosage of other medications you are taking may need to be reduced or other medications may need to be substituted.

DRUGS AND ALCOHOL

Alcohol is a potent drug all by itself, and you can be sure that it is going to affect many of the prescription and nonprescription medications that you may take as well. Alcohol is classified as a depressant drug. Its actions on body tissues are extremely complex, but in general, it will depress body functions. Should you take a tranquilizer along with alcohol, the sedative effect of the tranquilizer will be heightened by the alcohol and you are vulnerable to a drug interaction that can be life threatening, causing unconsciousness, illness, accidents, and inability to respond to emergencies.

Not only sedatives, but also antihistamines (allergy and cold medications) can be affected by alcohol use. Pain relievers, heart medications, and many other drugs interact with alcohol. Read all warning labels carefully and always ask your doctor or pharmacist if you plan to take alcohol, no matter how small the amount, while taking any drug.

A WORK OF CAUTION ABOUT DRUGS AND PREGNANCY

The best advice concerning taking drugs during pregnancy is **DON'T**, unless they are prescribed by your physician. Remember that your obstetrician may not know about the drugs that have been prescribed by another physician, a dentist, or any other health professional you may be consulting. It is important that you let your obstetrician know of all drugs you are taking, no matter how unimportant they may seem to be. This includes vitamins and home remedies. Your doctor may prescribe iron, vitamin, or calcium supplements while you are pregnant. He or she is the best source for information about your own necessity for taking these vitamins and for the appropriate dosages.

Because drugs have varying degrees of ability to penetrate the placenta and enter the bloodstream of the embryo or fetus, and because not everything is known about the action of drugs on the unborn baby, you should always assume that *any* drug you take will affect your baby, unless you are told otherwise by your doctor. Don't forget that alcohol is a drug as well and can cause fetal alcohol syndrome in the newborn, a lifelong impairment. The nicotine found in cigarette smoke is also a drug. If you are pregnant, consult your doctor before taking *anything*.

SOME DO'S AND DON'TS WHEN YOU ARE TAKING MEDICATION

- Give your doctor complete information about your medical condition, any drugs you are taking, and all sensitivities and allergies you know about to the best of your ability.

- Educate yourself about all drugs before you take them. Don't be afraid to ask questions of your doctor or insist that he or she clarify facts or issues you don't understand.
- Stay in touch with your doctor while you are on any medication; let him know at once of any unusual reactions you are having.
- Always be sure of the medicine you are taking. Read the label before you take it, since many drugs are packaged similarly.
- Store all your medicines away from moisture and heat.
- Don't change the amount of your dosage without first checking with your doctor and pharmacist.
- Don't use over-the-counter medications while you are taking a prescription drug without first checking with your doctor or pharmacist.
- Shake all liquid medicines before taking them.
- Do not freeze a drug that is to be refrigerated as this may affect the potency of the drug.
- Make sure you use a standard measuring spoon that you can get from your pharmacist. Teaspoons and tablespoons are not accurate enough.
- Follow all special instructions when taking medication, such as taking on an empty or full stomach.
- If you have food allergies or hay fever or other allergies, let your doctor know. They may predispose you to allergies to certain medications.
- If you are planning surgery, let your doctor know all of the medicines you have taken recently. Some medicines may remain in the system even after you feel they have worn off long ago, and may interact with your surgical medications.
- Store all drugs out of the reach of children. Have the number of your local poison control center close by.
- If you are pregnant, take only those medications prescribed by your doctor and never use alcohol, cocaine, psychedelics, or other mood-altering drugs.

- If you are seeing more than one doctor, make sure all doctors know what the other doctors have been prescribing.
- Don't save leftover medications to take another time. Always take the medication prescribed according to instruction. Discard all leftover medication. Some medications lose potency past the expiration date, but other medicines can change their chemical state and actually become toxic.
- Make sure medicines that you dispose of are out of the reach of children and pets.
- If you need a refill, call your doctor.
- If the drug causes drowsiness, be especially careful when driving or operating machinery.
- Be aware that many drugs filter through to the breast milk of a nursing mother. If you are nursing a child, do not take any drug without first checking with your doctor.

CHAPTER VII

Guide to Drugs Available by Mail-Order Import

This chapter provides a basic overview of many popular drugs that are available by mail order through the sources listed in Appendix I of this book. The chapter is presented for information purposes only. It is not intended as a complete guide to all drugs on the market, nor is it intended to offer any kind of recommendation for usage or ordering purposes.

It should be noted that I have only included information about drugs that meet FDA and DEA requirements for legal importation. This is true even where there is a hint of a possible question about whether or not a given drug is legal for import. For example, there is a small amount of DEA controlled narcotic or narcotic derivatives in both Lomotil and aspirin with codeine. These drugs appear to fall outside the scope of laws pertaining to DEA controlled substances; but I couldn't get anyone in the DEA to say this for sure, so I left them out to be on the safe side.

(Let me give you an interesting aside here. One DEA official who I talked to about this problem said, "You never know about things like this. Technically, the law says that a person can be punished with a sentence of up to eighteen months in jail if convicted for the illegal import of codeine. Who knows how the courts might rule on this!" I replied, "I can't believe that the DEA doesn't have more important issues on its hands, like cocaine and crack for example." He responded, "You would think so. However, during the Nixon administration that wasn't always the case." That was enough for me. I wouldn't take a chance on these drugs, and I don't think you should either.)

The main purpose of this chapter is to provide a brief reference for those who want a quick explanation of the uses, side effects, and dosages of just those drugs that are available from the mail-order sources listed in Appendix I. It is not intended as a total drug information compendium.

Before using any of these medications it is strongly recommended that you consult your physician, as well as more authoritative sources such as the latest yearly editions of the *Physicians' Desk Reference* and *Drug Facts and Comparisons*. To find out more information about drugs manufactured outside the US, refer to *The Pharmacological Basis of Therapeutics* and *Martindale: The Extra Pharmacopoeia*. Complete reference material is given in the Bibliography.

Note: Because the brand names of the various drugs differ from country to country, the drugs in this chapter are organized alphabetically by generic name, in most cases. The exceptions are where combinations of ingredients are involved. In these cases, the listing is by brand name. Also, for interest's sake, I have included a few "home remedies" that are popular in other countries. These are listed by brand name. Brand names are indicated with an asterisk.

ACETAZOLAMIDE

Acetazolamide is a diuretic, used in managing swelling, glaucoma, epilepsy, mountain sickness, muscular and respiratory disorders, and sleep apnea. It is also an anticonvulsant that is sometimes used for petit mal seizures in children and for cases of acute mountain climbing sickness.

How Acetazolamide Works

Acetazolamide is of the sulfa family and lessens the body's production of a chemical called carbonic anhydrase. It causes increased excretion of sodium, potassium, and chloride in the urine.

Recommended Dosage

The normal dosage in adults is 250 milligrams to 1 gram daily, usually in divided doses of 250 milligrams. Amounts over 1 gram don't seem to increase the effect.

Side Effects of Acetazolamide

Reported side effects have included malaise or "feeling sick," fatigue, depression, excitement, headache, weight loss, and gastrointestinal disturbances. Drowsiness, numbness, and tingling of the face and hands have also been reported. Acetazolamide can give rise to kidney stones and other kidney abnormalities. Fever, thirst, dizziness, ataxia, nearsightedness (temporary), ringing in the ears, and other hearing disturbances have also been reported.

People who have sodium or potassium depletion should not use this drug, as it may worsen that condition. It may also aggravate conditions such as kidney impairment, Addison's disease, or certain types of glaucoma. Pregnant women should avoid taking it in the first trimester of pregnancy. People with diabetes should take this drug with care.

ALLOPURINOL

Allopurinol is used in the treatment of uric acid disorders resulting in gout, recurrent stone formation, kidney disorders, enzyme and blood disorders, and in cancer therapy. Allopurinol is not used to treat an acute attack of gout, and when taken during an acute attack, may prolong the illness. Although allopurinol is not used to treat acute gout, it may prevent attacks. In treating recurrent gout, the objective is to reduce the overproduction of uric acid which leads to painful deposits of monosodium urate in the joints and soft tissues.

How Allopurinol Works

Allopurinol diminishes the body's production of uric acid in people experiencing gout. This results in lower concentrations of uric acid in the blood and the urine so that monosodium urate deposits are discouraged from forming.

Recommended Dosage

The usual dose of allopurinol necessary to reduce the possibility of gout attacks is 100 milligrams daily, by mouth initially. This dose is increased as necessary until the concentration of uric acid is at acceptable levels.

Side Effects of Allopurinol

The most common side effect of allopurinol is a rash, which may occur more frequently in people with kidney failure. Other signs of allergy may be fever or chills that could lead to kidney failure. Other side effects include peripheral neuralgia, loss of hair, nausea, vomiting, stomach pain, drowsiness, and vertigo. During the first few months of treatment, the gout condition may actually become worse. People taking anticoagulants or diuretics should be carefully monitored.

AMIKACIN SULFATE

Amikacin sulfate was developed from an antibiotic called kanamycin and is related to the gentamycin family of antibiotics. It is used in the treatment of severe gram-negative infections. This term refers to a diagnostic test taken to determine what kind of bacterial infection you have. Amikacin sulfate is usually reserved to treat infections which have been resistant to other antibiotics such as gentamycin and tobramycin. As with gentamycin, amikacin may be used in conjunction with penicillins and with cephalosporins.

Infections which this antibiotic has been used to treat include meningitis, osteomyelitis, septicemia, tuberculosis, and urinary tract infections, among others.

How Amikacin Works

Amikacin is called a semisynthetic aminoglycoside antibiotic. This family of drugs works by interfering chemically with the bacteria's use of protein. Amikacin is effective against many types of bacteria and is a broad spectrum antibiotic. It is very active in breaking down the defenses of the bacteria. Some hospitals have restricted their use of this drug in order to prevent the development of resistant strains of bacteria.

Recommended Dosage

The recommended dose is 15 milligrams of amikacin per kilogram of body weight, divided into two or three equal portions. People who have kidney failure should take a smaller dosage.

Side Effects of Amikacin

All antibiotics of this family may produce side effects that can result in permanent hearing loss (ototoxicity). Ototoxicity has also been reported by people who apply this family of drugs, including neomycin, to their skin, especially if they apply it to a large vulnerable area, such as a large burn. Previous exposure or sensitivity may also be a factor.

People using this drug have also experienced kidney problems, which are reversible when they stop taking amikacin. People with kidney failure are especially at risk for severe reactions, so use of this drug should be carefully supervised by a physician. Difficulty in breathing and muscular paralysis have also been reported.

Do not mix aminoglycosides, such as amikacin, and penicillins in the same bottle, because the penicillin will inactivate the aminoglycoside. Amikacin may interact with frusemide and other diuretics, indomethacin, heparin, cisplatin, and may interfere with certain diagnostic tests. It should not be used by people with myasthenia gravis. Those who are receiving other drugs with a neuromuscular blocking agent must also exercise caution in using amikacin.

AMOXICILLIN

Amoxicillin is used to treat a large number of infections and diseases caused by both gram-positive and gram-negative microorganisms. It has been used successfully to treat ear, strep, intestinal, mouth, and respiratory tract infections, such as bronchitis and pneumonia, tonsil infections, venereal infections, and many others. It is not considered effective against staph infections.

Amoxicillin is a member of the penicillin family, one of the most important of the antibiotics. Ever since readily available penicillin was developed in the 1940s there have been many variations and synthetic versions of its basic chemical structure.

How Amoxicillin Works

Penicillin works by preventing the cell wall of the bacteria from functioning properly, thus destroying the entire cell. Amoxicillin is considered a broad-spectrum antibiotic, meaning that it destroys a great variety of different organisms.

Recommended Dosage

Amoxicillin is rapidly and completely absorbed when taken by mouth, and food does not interfere with its action. The common dosage for adults is 250 milligrams every eight hours; for children 20 milligrams per kilogram of body weight per day in divided doses every eight hours.

These dosages may be increased to 500 milligrams every eight hours for adults and 40 milligrams per kilogram per day in divided doses every eight hours for children. Children who weigh over 20 kilograms should be given the appropriate adult dosage, and never a dosage exceeding that for an adult.

Side Effects of Amoxicillin

People who are allergic to penicillin should not use amoxicillin, as there is a danger of a massive allergic (anaphylactic) reaction which can be life threatening. Some people develop skin rashes or even severe lesions when exposed to penicillin. People who have infectious mononucleosis develop rashes after receiving penicillin. Other reactions include fever, bronchial spasm, serum sickness, dermatitis, nephritis, and Stevens-Johnson syndrome. Most symptoms clear up rapidly once the drug is removed, but severe allergic reactions have been known to result in death.

AMPICILLIN

Ampicillin is used to treat all varieties of infections, including bronchial, venereal, cardiac, respiratory, urinary and gastrointestinal, strep, and many others. Ampicillin is ineffective for most staph infections.

How Ampicillin Works

Ampicillin works like other members of the penicillin family by penetrating the outer cell wall of the bacterium and binding to certain proteins that are essential to maintaining the cell wall's integrity. Like amoxicillin, ampicillin is a synthetic penicillin that is effective against most gram-positive and some gram-negative bacterial infections.

Recommended Dosage

The dosage varies according to the type and severity of the infection, the patient's age, and kidney function. For mild to severe infections, the usual adult (people weighing over 44 kilograms) dosage is 2 to 4 grams per day, given at six-hour intervals. For people weighing less than 44 kilograms, the indication is 100 milligrams per kilogram per day in equally divided doses at six- to eight-hour intervals.

For infections of the gastrointestinal and urinary tract, people weighing over 44 kilograms should receive 500 milligrams every six hours; those weighing less than 44 kilograms should receive 100 milligrams per kilogram per day in equally divided doses at six- to eight-hour intervals.

Side Effects of Ampicillin

If you must take this drug for a long period of time, your kidney and liver function should be tested and evaluated. Occasional severe allergic reactions have occurred when people use this antibiotic, and it should not be taken if you have a history of hypersensitivity to penicillin. The possibility of developing suprainfections or penicillin-resistant infections should be kept in mind when using this drug.

ATENOLOL

Atenolol is one of a class of drugs called beta blockers, used in the treatment of high blood pressure, angina pectoris, cardiac arrhythmias, tachycardia (rapid heartbeat); it is also prescribed to lessen the body's responses to adrenaline and isoprenaline and to combat anxiety. Beta blockers may reduce the risk of a second heart attack and moderate some of the effects of anxiety. Beta blockers also reduce eye pressure and are sometimes used in treating glaucoma.

How Atenolol Works

Atenolol reduces stress on the heart by lessening the stimulation that comes from various body chemicals. Atenolol diminishes the rate and force of the heart's contractions, and decreases the rate at which the impulses that stimulate the heart travel through the system. This reduces the response of the heart to stress and exercise. It also lowers blood pressure in people with hypertension, while at the same time raising the tolerance of the heart to exercise.

Recommended Dosage

Atenolol is usually given by mouth in the treatment of high blood pressure, in amounts of 100 milligrams daily as a single dose, although some patients may respond to 50 milligrams. The usual dose for angina pectoris is 50 to 100 milligrams daily, given as single or divided doses.

Side Effects of Atenolol

Atenolol has few serious problems associated with its use. The most common side effects are headache, dizziness and light-headedness, fatigue, weakness, nausea, slowed heartbeat, edema, diarrhea, depression, dyspnea (difficulty in breathing), anxiety, chest pain, lethargy, drowsiness, and malaise, or a feeling of illness.

Rare side effects may include Raynaud's phenomenon, cold hands and feet, hallucinations, psychotic episodes, disturbances of sleep and vision. Loss of hearing, paresthesia, bronchospasm, blood disorder, and skin rashes are other reported side effects as are fluid retention, allergic responses, and dry eyes.

This drug should not be given to people who have bronchospasm or other obstructive airway disease, metabolic acidosis, slowed heartbeat or partial heart block or congestive heart failure. It may mask the symptoms of hyperthyroidism or of hypoglycemia in patients with diabetes mellitus.

ATROPINE SULFATE

Atropine is used to relieve spasms of the gastrointestinal tract and to treat colic and gastric and duodenal ulcers. It reduces tremor and muscular rigidity in Parkinson's disease. Since it increases the heart rate, it is often used during cardiopulmonary resuscitation or to correct a slow heartbeat. It is also used before surgery to reduce salivary and bronchial secretions.

How Atropine Works

Atropine is of a class of medications called antimuscarinic alkaloids, which has complex effects on the central and peripheral nervous systems. It first stimulates then depresses the central nervous system. It also has antispasmodic actions on smooth muscle tissue. It also reduces secretions, especially saliva and bronchial secretions, as well as perspiration.

Recommended Dosage

Consult your physician, because dosages vary depending upon purpose and condition of health.

Side Effects of Atropine

Side effects include dryness of the mouth, difficulty in talking and swallowing, thirst, dilation of the pupils, flushing and dryness of the skin; slow followed by rapid heartbeat, palpitations, arrhythmias; and urinary urgency, difficulty, and retention. Constipation may result and also occasional vomiting, giddiness, and staggering.

This drug may lead to retention of urine in men with enlarged prostates, and is contraindicated in cases of pyloric stenosis or paralytic ileus. In people with ulcerative colitis, its use may lead to ileus or megacolon. Those with closed-angle glaucoma should not take this drug, since it may raise intraocular pressure. Other precautions include people with myasthenia gravis, tachycardia, heart attack, and cardiac insufficiency or failure.

Using Atropine in Combination with Other Drugs

The effects of this drug and other drugs with atropine may be enhanced by taking drugs with antimuscarinic effects, such as amantadine, some antihistamines, butyrophenones, and phenothiazines, as well as tricyclic antidepressants. The reduction in motility of the intestines may affect the absorption of other drugs.

AUGMENTIN*

Augmentin is the brand name for a mixture of clavulanic acid and the antibiotic amoxicillin, which has been useful for urinary tract infections that have been resistant to other methods of treatment. Augmentin has also been used to treat middle ear infections, bronchial infections, lung infections, septicemia, and sexually transmitted diseases.

How Augmentin Works

See Amoxicillin. Clavulanic acid resembles penicillin, but has some important chemical differences. It has the ability to penetrate the cell walls of bacteria and inactivate some of their enzymes, thus destroying them. Consequently, it enhances the activity of various antibiotics such as penicillin.

Recommended Dosage

Consult your physician. Augmentin is given as a ratio of the amoxicillin to the clavulanic acid, usually two or four parts amoxicillin to one part clavulanic acid.

Side Effects of Augmentin

See Amoxicillin.

BENDROFLUMETHIAZIDE

Bendroflumethiazide belongs to the thiazide family of diuretics. It is used to help the body release water in the treatment of edema, heart disorders, and high blood pressure. It is also used to suppress production of breast milk and to reduce the possibility of stroke. Bendroflumethiazide may also be recommended for controlling premenstrual fluid retention and preventing the formation of kidney stones.

How Bendroflumethiazide Works

The thiazide family of diuretics are chemically related to the sulfa drugs and work in the kidneys to help the body get rid of excess salt, as well as other elements.

Recommended Dosage

The action of bendroflumethiazide begins about two hours after taking it, and lasts for about twelve to eighteen hours. For edema, the initial dose is 5 to 10 milligrams daily or on alternate days. In some cases, initial doses of up to 20 milligrams may be required. Maintenance doses range from 2.5 to 10 milligrams daily or on intermittent days.

In treating hypertension, the treatment is 2.5 to 5 milligrams daily, either alone or in conjunction with other hypertensive drugs. If treatment is to be prolonged, supplements of potassium may also be prescribed.

Side Effects of Bendroflumethiazide

There are many imbalances that may occur from the increased excretion of urine. Signs of electrolyte imbalance include dry mouth, thirst, weakness, lethargy, drowsiness, restlessness, muscle pain and cramps, and gastrointestinal disturbances. Other side effects of bendroflumethiazide may include loss of appetite, stomach irritation, nausea, vomiting, constipation or diarrhea, impotence, yellow vision, skin rashes, sensitivity to light, fluid in the lungs, and jaundice.

Bendroflumethiazide and all other diuretics may cause a disturbance in the metabolism, such as hyperglycemia or glycosuria in the diabetic. The use of digitalis or other heart medications may have to be suspended while someone is taking these diuretics. People with severe coronary artery disease or cirrhosis of the liver need to be carefully watched by their physician while taking this drug.

BISACODYL

Bisacodyl is a common laxative useful in the treatment of constipation and in helping to empty the bowel before diagnostic tests. It is frequently used by people with spinal cord injuries, also to evacuate the bowel. Bisacodyl is active mainly in the large intestine and takes effect within six to twelve hours of administration.

How Bisacodyl Works

Bisacodyl works by stimulating the accumulation of water and electrolytes in the wall of the intestine. It also enhances intestinal movement. Both of these actions expedite transit of the contents of the colon.

Recommended Dosage

Bisacodyl is usually given in 10 milligram doses daily, administered at night. Doses of up to 30 milligrams have been given for complete emptying of the bowel.

Side Effects of Bisacodyl

Although bisacodyl tablets are coated to help avoid stomach irritation, stomach discomfort—such as colic or cramps—is often reported. Prolonged use or overdose may result in diarrhea with loss of water and electrolytes, especially potassium. There is also a possibility of the colon losing its function from overuse of bisacodyl.

This drug should not be given to people who have intestinal obstructions, undiagnosed stomach pain, or other symptoms. People with inflammatory bowel disease should take this only under the guidance of their physician.

BONJELA ANTISEPTIC ORAL GEL*

Bonjela is a topical analgesic ointment useful in relief of teething pain and other mouth sores.

How Bonjela Works

The active ingredient in bonjela is choline salicylate, a compound with similar qualities to aspirin.

Recommended Dosage

Follow the directions on the package and apply to teeth and gums to relieve the pain of mouth lesions.

Side Effects of Bonjela

Precautions should be used in children, as the active ingredient can be absorbed through the skin. Discontinue use if dizziness, nausea, or headache are present. Do not use on children if fever or other flu symptoms are present, as there is a risk of Reye's syndrome, a serious disease characterized by stupor and dullness.

BUFLOMEDIL HYDROCHLORIDE

Buflomedil is a vasodilator, meaning that it opens up or expands the blood vessels. It has been used in the treatment of peripheral artery disease, where there is cramplike pain due to an insufficient blood supply. It has oxygen-sparing activity and may help prevent blood clots.

In people with cerebrovascular disease, buflomedil helps to improve their coordination and reasoning functions. It has been reported by one source to be as effective or more effective than ergot alkaloids in helping elderly people who have become senile from having too little oxygen-bearing blood entering their brain.

Encouraging preliminary results have also been obtained using buflomedil to treat Raynaud's phenomenon, diabetic retinopathy, frostbite, pains related to growing, and vestibular disorders of the inner ear. This drug is still under study to determine its full therapeutic value, but results so far have confirmed that it is of significant value in treating the above conditions.

How Buflomedil Works

Buflomedil's main beneficial property seems to be an improvement in the nutritional blood flow in ischemic tissues without having overall systemic effects.

Recommended Dosage

The usual dosage is by mouth, in amounts of 450 milligrams daily. This dosage should be divided into three equal amounts throughout the day.

Side Effects of Buflomedil

Buflomedil has been reported to cause gastrointestinal disturbances, headache, hypotension, and paresthesia. High doses may produce severe hypotension, tachycardia, and convulsions. Overdose may result in convulsions, especially in people with impaired kidney function and low body weight.

CAPTOPRIL

Captopril is a relatively new drug, used to lower high blood pressure. It is often taken with a diuretic drug to control water retention. The effect of taking captopril is usually a rapid lowering of blood pressure, usually within about one and one-half hours. Captopril is used when other drugs are not suitable or have produced side effects. It is also used in the treatment of congestive heart failure.

How Captopril Works

Captopril works by preventing the conversion of a powerful hormone called angiotensin I into angiotensin II. This hormone influences the production of other hormones that regulate blood pressure. Studies have shown that captopril increases cardiac output and reduces arterial blood pressure, vascular resistance, and pulmonary blood pressure.

Recommended Dosage

The initial recommended dosage of captopril is 12.5 milligrams twice daily by mouth, increased gradually if necessary, to gain optimum response. To control mild to moderate hypertension, the usual dose is 25 milligrams or 50 milligrams twice daily. For severe hypertension, a dose of 50 milligrams three times daily should not be exceeded.

In the treatment of congestive heart failure, the initial dose ranges between 6.25 and 12.5 milligrams under close medical supervision. The usual maintenance dose is 25 milligrams three times daily. When possible, diuretics should be stopped before giving captopril initially.

People who have congestive heart failure and who have been taking diuretics may experience very low blood pressure when taking captopril. This undesirable effect can be minimized by taking a very low dose, preferably before bedtime.

Side Effects of Captopril

One of the side effects of captopril is a sense of well-being, which was thought to be drug-induced euphoria, but which may come from being able to stop other drugs. The full benefits often take as long as several weeks to be realized.

Captopril should be used with great caution by people who have kidney impairment, particularly if renovascular disease is suspected. These people should be monitored closely for protein in their urine. People with lupus or scleroderma should take captopril only under close medical supervision and with great caution. Regular white blood cell counts should be taken.

Avoid strenuous exercise in very hot weather, as this may cause water loss and a consequent sudden drop in blood pressure. This drug may cause dizziness if you rise quickly after sitting or lying down.

Using Captopril in Combination with Other Drugs

The drug indomethacin has been shown to reduce or abolish the therapeutic effect of captopril. Captopril will have an additive effect when used with other diuretics. Beta-adrenergic drugs may increase the blood pressure–lowering ability of captopril. Avoid over-the-counter cough and cold remedies while taking captopril, except if prescribed by a physician.

CARBIMAZOLE

Carbimazole is an antithyroid drug which is most popular in the United Kingdom and Europe. It is used to control hyperthyroidism such as Graves' disease and also as a part of treatment for the life-threatening condition known as thyroid storm. Carbimazole has been used as a "growth promoter" in the feed of animals, but since it is capable of being passed to humans through the meat and by-products of these animals, the use of such agents is now banned.

How Carbimazole Works

Carbimazole works by limiting the formation of the thyroid hormone. It also has some immunosuppressive activity. Antithyroid agents such as carbimazole have a reversible effect on the thyroid gland.

Recommended Dosage

When used to control hyperthyroidism, carbimazole is usually given by mouth in an initial dosage of 30 to 60 milligrams daily in divided doses at eight-hour intervals, according to the severity of the condition. Improvement is usually seen in one to three weeks, with control of symptoms in one to three months. The dosage is then reduced to the smallest amount which can effectively control the disorder. Common maintenance doses are 5 to 15 milligrams daily.

Side Effects of Carbimazole

Side effects of carbimazole occur most commonly during the first two months of treatment. These may include nausea, fever, vomiting, sore throat, blood abnormalities, gastric distress, headache, and skin rashes, including urticaria and pruritus. Joint pain, leukopenia, and aplastic anemia have also been reported.

Antithyroid agents cross the placenta and may cause thyroid deficiency or goiter in the newborn. If blood disorders such as agranulocytosis or bone marrow depression occur, carbimazole should be withdrawn immediately, and if necessary, antibiotics and blood transfusions given.

CEFACLOR

Cefaclor is taken by mouth for the treatment of mild to moderate infections of the respiratory and urinary tracts or of the skin and the ear. For severe infections treatment by injection with cephalosporins is preferable.

Cefaclor belongs to the family of cephalosporin antibiotics, which were developed in 1948 from a fungus found growing in the sea near Sardinia. Cultures of this fungus were found to inhibit the growth of staphylococci, and to cure those infections and typhoid fever in man.

How Cefaclor Works

Cefaclor seems to act against the cell wall of bacteria, much like penicillin does. There have been so many derivatives of the cephalosporins that they are now classified by generations.

Recommended Dosage

The usual dose is 250 milligrams every eight hours, although up to 4 grams has been given. The usual dose for children is 20 milligrams per kilogram of body weight, which may be increased to 40 milligrams if necessary, but not exceeding a daily dose of 1 gram. Children over five years usually receive 250 milligrams three times daily; children one to five years 125 milligrams three times daily; under one year, 62.5 milligrams three times daily.

Side Effects of Cefaclor

Side effects can include nausea, vomiting, diarrhea, and abdominal discomfort. Allergic reactions such as skin rashes, urticaria, edema, and anaphylaxis could also occur, as well as suprainfections with resistant microorganisms.

About 10 percent of people who are allergic to penicillin are also thought to be allergic to the cephalosporins, so care must be taken by these people in using the cephalosporins. Each variety of cephalosporin has a different range of effectiveness, although many overlap.

CEFATRIZINE

Cefatrizine is another member of the cephalosporin family of antibiotics, and is similar to cephalexin. When taken by mouth, it is considered effective against certain strains of bacteria, including *Enterobacter*, *Hemophilus*, and *Proteus*. It is used in infections of the genitourinary tract, respiratory tract, and skin.

How Cefatrizine Works

Cefatrizine works very well when taken by mouth. It exits the body by means of the kidney, so people with impaired or reduced kidney function must be careful with this drug. Each member of the cephalosporin family works best with certain infections, so it is important to seek the guidance of your physician in deciding which to take.

Recommended Dosage

Cefatrizine is given by mouth in doses up to 3 grams daily. Dosage and length of treatment will depend upon the type and severity of the infection. The usual dose for adults is 1 to 2 grams daily given in divided doses at six-, eight-, or twelve-hour intervals. For infants and children, consult your physician.

Side Effects of Cefatrizine

Adverse reactions are generally considered mild, however this, like other antibiotics can provoke allergic reactions ranging from skin rashes to anaphylaxis.

CEPHALEXIN

Cephalexin is an antibiotic used to treat infections of the respiratory tract, urinary tract, and skin as well as ear infections and other responsive infections.

How Cephalexin Works

Cephalexin is usually taken by mouth. It is almost completely absorbed from the gastrointestinal tract and is widely distributed throughout the body. It has been used to treat pregnant women for urinary infections.

Recommended Dosage

Cephalexin is usually given to adults in 1 to 2 gram daily doses, at six-, eight-, or twelve-hour intervals. For severe or deep-seated infections the dose may be increased to 6 grams daily, but the use of an injection should be then considered. Infants and children can be given 25 milligrams to 100 milligrams per kilogram of body weight in divided doses up to a maximum of 4 grams daily. Children aged five to twelve years may receive 250 milligrams three times daily; aged one to five years 125 milligrams three times daily; under one year, 125 milligrams twice daily.

Side Effects of Cephalexin

This drug can cause side effects including nausea, vomiting, diarrhea, and stomach discomfort. Allergic reactions include skin rashes, urticaria, eosinophilia, angioedema, and massive anaphylactic reaction in severe allergies. A rise in liver enzyme values may occur as well as suprainfections of resistant organisms such as candida. If you know or suspect that you may be allergic to cephalosporins, you should not use this drug. About 10 percent of people allergic to penicillin will also be allergic to cephalosporins.

CHLORPHENIRAMINE

Chlorpheniramine is an antihistamine used to relieve the symptoms of seasonal allergies, sneezing, runny, itching nose, and red eyes. It is sometimes used in conjunction with other drugs to reduce congestion and coughing. The sedative effects may be useful in treatment for motion sickness.

How Chlorpheniramine Works

Antihistamines work by blocking the undesirable effects of some of the body's natural chemicals, called histamines.

Recommended Dosage

Chlorpheniramine is usually given in dosages of 4 milligrams three to four times daily. For children, consult your physician.

Side Effects of Chlorpheniramine

Antihistamines should not be given to premature infants, newborns, or people with glaucoma, urinary retention, or prostate disease. Antihistamines should not be used during acute asthma attacks.

Using Chlorpheniramine in Combination with Other Drugs

Antihistamines enhance the effects of other drugs such as alcohol, barbiturates, hypnotics, narcotics of any kind, sedatives, tranquilizers, and antidepressants. Antihistamines may cause drowsiness, so care should be used in operating automobiles or machinery.

CIMETIDINE

Cimetidine is used for the short-term treatment of duodenal and gastric ulcer, esophageal reflux, persistent indigestion, and the secretion of too much stomach acid. Cimetidine has revolutionized the treatment of ulcers, proving to be quite safe and effective. It is sometimes used for gastrointestinal bleeding, to reduce malabsorption and fluid loss in people with short bowel syndrome, and in cases of pancreatic insufficiency. Treatment with a reduced dose of cimetidine is also considered valuable to prevent recurrence of healed ulcers.

How Cimetidine Works

Cimetidine lowers the amounts of gastric acid secreted, both during the day and at night, and also inhibits the amount of acids stimulated by food and caffeine. Drugs of this type are called histamine H_2 receptor antagonists.

Recommended Dosage

When cimetidine is given by mouth, the dosages should generally be taken with meals. The usual dose is 800 milligrams twice daily, 400 milligrams in the morning and 400 milligrams at bedtime. Other regimens are 200 milligrams or, if necessary, 400 milligrams three times daily with 400 milligrams at bedtime.

In the management of gastric and duodenal ulcers, a single daily dose of 800 milligrams may be given by mouth at bedtime. This dose is continued for four weeks in the case of duodenal ulcers and six weeks for gastric ulcers. When indicated, a maintenance dose of 400 milligrams may be given at bedtime, or once in the morning and once at bedtime.

Side Effects of Cimetidine

Cimetidine is relatively free of side effects, with the most commonly reported ones being diarrhea, dizziness, fatigue, and rashes. Older people may experience confusion, which is reversible. A possibility of impotence in men has also been reported.

Using Cimetidine in Combination with Other Drugs

Cimetidine has been known to interact with or affect the function of other drugs, including anticoagulants, phenytoin, and diazepam. Before taking cimetidine, the underlying conditions causing the need should be evaluated by a physician, as the drug may mask the symptoms of malignancy and delay diagnosis.

CLONIDINE HYDROCHLORIDE

Clonidine hydrochloride is used in the treatment of high blood pressure of all grades, although there are less active and toxic drugs now available. It is also used to prevent migraine headaches and to reduce menopausal hot flashes, as well as in treating the symptoms of opiate withdrawal and Tourette's syndrome.

How Clonidine Hydrochloride Works

Clonidine hydrochloride appears to act by stimulating certain hormone receptors in the brain and causing the dilation or expansion of the blood vessels, thereby decreasing blood pressure dramatically, often within one hour.

Recommended Dosage

The usual dosage in treating hypertension is one-tenth of a milligram twice a day, which may be raised by your physician until maximum control is established. The dose must be tailored to the patient's individual needs. At no time should a person be taking more than 2.4 milligrams per day.

Some people develop a tolerance to clonidine hydrochloride. When this happens, blood pressure will increase, necessitating a change in dosage or in the drug. Clonidine hydrochloride is not recommended for women who are pregnant or who plan to become pregnant.

Side Effects of Clonidine Hydrochloride

Possible side effects include dry mouth, drowsiness, sedation, constipation, dizziness, headache, and fatigue. Other adverse side effects may include loss of appetite, a feeling of illness, nausea, vomiting, weight gain, breast enlargement, changes in the heart, strange dreams or nightmares, difficulty sleeping, nervousness, restlessness, anxiety, depression, rash, hives, itching, thinning of the hair, difficulty in urinating, impotence, and dryness and burning of the eyes.

Abrupt withdrawal of the drug can cause severe reactions. People who stop taking clonidine hydrochloride suddenly may experience an abrupt rise in blood pressure, agitation, headache, and nervousness. These effects can be reversed by starting the drug again or taking another antihypertensive drug.

Using Clonidine Hydrochloride in Combination with Other Drugs

Clonidine hydrochloride is a depressant and will enhance the effect of alcohol, barbiturates, sedatives, and tranquilizers. These should all be avoided. Antidepressant drugs may counteract the effects of clonidine hydrochloride. This drug should never be prescribed with a beta-blocking agent.

93

CLOTRIMAZOLE

Clotrimazole is used in the treatment of candidiasis infections, tinea, and pityriasis versicolor. It is also used for vaginal infections.

How Clotrimazole Works

Clotrimazole is an antifungal agent that has action against many common infections. It works by helping to break down the cell wall of the fungus and destroying it.

Recommended Dosage

Clotrimazole cream is applied to the skin affected by fungus infections or used as directed by the physician.

Side Effects of Clotrimazole

When applied topically, adverse reactions have included irritation and burning or allergic contact dermatitis.

CLOXACILLIN SODIUM

Cloxacillin sodium is a penicillin used to treat infections that are resistant to benzylpenicillin, including infections of the skin and soft tissues, bones and joints, respiratory tract, urinary tract, middle ear, heart, blood, and brain. It is also used for streptococcus infections and staph infections that are resistant to other types of penicillins. Cloxacillin sodium can prevent infections during major operations, especially in heart and bone surgery.

How Cloxacillin Sodium Works

Cloxacillin sodium works by inhibiting the growth of most penicillinase-producing staphylococci. For that reason, it is not a substitute for other members of the penicillin family in most cases. Cloxacillins are the best choice for infections that are less vulnerable to other families of antibiotics.

Recommended Dosage

For adults the recommended dose is 250 to 500 milligrams taken four times daily one hour before or two hours after meals. Children under ten take half the adult dose.

Side Effects of Cloxacillin Sodium

Such complications as agranulocytosis, jaundice, phlebitis, eye problems, angioedema, or bronchospasm may occur. A sensitivity reaction may produce urticaria, joint pain, fever, eosinophilia, skin rashes, anemia, and leukopenia. If you are allergic to penicillin, you may also be allergic to cloxacillin sodium. Convulsions and other signs of toxicity may occur with very high doses, particularly in people who have impaired kidneys. Blood and liver dysfunctions may also occur, as well as diarrhea, nausea, and heartburn.

This drug may interact with probenecid, and may interfere with some urinary glucose or blood protein tests.

DICLOFENAC

Diclofenac is an antirheumatic drug used for relief in the treatment of the pain and inflammation of arthritis and rheumatoid arthritis, ankylosing spondylitis, acute gout, and following some surgical procedures.

How Diclofenac Works

Diclofenac works by inhibiting prostaglandin synthesis. That gives it anti-inflammatory and pain-relieving qualities.

Recommended Dosage

For adults, diclofenac is given 75 to 150 milligrams daily in divided doses. The recommended dose for children is 1 to 3 milligrams per kilogram of body weight daily in divided doses.

Side Effects of Diclofenac

The most frequent adverse effects are gastrointestinal disturbances, such as peptic ulcers and gastrointestinal bleeding. Other reported side effects are headache, dizziness, rashes, nervousness, pruritis, edema, depression, blurred vision, abnormality of liver function tests, and kidney impairment.

This medication should be given with extra care to people with asthma or bronchospasm, bleeding disorders, cardiovascular disease, kidney impairment, or to those receiving anticoagulants. Diclofenac may interact with digoxin and lithium. People with aspirin sensitivity are capable of developing reactions to diclofenac.

DIETHYLAMINE SALICYLATE 10 PERCENT

This cream is considered useful in the relief of muscle aches and strains, and in lessening the discomforts of arthritis and rheumatism. As a salicylate-based ointment, it utilizes the inflammation and pain-relieving properties of aspirin.

How Diethylamine Works

Aspirin has pain-relieving and anti-inflammatory qualities, used in the relief of less severe types of pain, such as headaches and joint and muscle pain and in chronic inflammatory disorders such as arthritis.

Recommended Dosage

Follow the instructions on the label; massage into the affected area gently, and repeat when necessary. This medication should not be taken internally or used in the eye area.

Side Effects of Diethylamine

The same cautions apply to this as to other aspirin-related medications. This drug may be absorbed through the skin, so it should not be used by people who know they are allergic to aspirin or other salicylates. Because of the possibility of Reye's syndrome, diethylamine should not be given to children under twelve. Repeated administration of large doses may cause ringing of the ears, dizziness, sweating, nausea, confusion, headaches, vomiting, and hypoglycemia.

DIMETHICONE

Dimethicone is used for the treatment of stomach gas and flatulence and to relieve abdominal distension and dyspepsia caused by air or foam in the intestinal tract. It is also used postoperatively to relieve minor gas symptoms.

How Dimethicone Works

Dimethicone works by using a fine silicone dioxide to reduce the surface tension of gas bubbles in the stomach, causing them to break apart.

Recommended Dosage

Doses of up to 2 grams daily are used, often in conjunction with an antacid.

Side Effects of Dimethicone

Used over a long period of time, silicate-based products may result in the development of silicate kidney stones.

DIPYRIDAMOLE

Dipyridamole is an anticoagulant, antithrombotic, antiplatelet drug, used to prevent blood clots in people who have had heart surgery or kidney transplants. It is also used to widen blood vessels for long-term management of angina pectoris and to help prevent strokes.

How Dipyridamole Works

This drug works by inhibiting certain chemical functions that must take place before blood can clot. Dipyridamole is sometimes given in conjunction with aspirin and is being investigated for use in the treatment of stroke. When it is used to treat angina, dipyridamole increases the supply of blood to the heart and thus provides the heart with an increase of oxygen.

Recommended Dosage

The usual dose is 100 milligrams four times daily before food, increased if necessary to 600 milligrams daily, often in conjunction with aspirin or another anticoagulant. When used as a vasodilator in long-term management of angina pectoris, dipyridamole is given in doses of 50 milligrams three times daily.

Side Effects of Dipyridamole

Adverse effects of this drug include gastric disturbances, nausea, vomiting, diarrhea, headache, dizziness, faintness, flushing, and skin rash. Dipyridamole should be given with care to people with hypotension and should not be given to those with hemodynamic instability following a heart attack. Taking other anticoagulant drugs at the same time may result in excessive bleeding.

FAMOTIDINE

Famotidine is used for the relief and management of gastric and duodenal ulcers, for esophageal reflux, persistent indigestion, for those who have experienced stomach bleeding, and to reduce malabsorption and fluid loss through the intestine. It is one of a relatively new class of drugs that has changed the treatment of stomach ulcer, shortening the time for healing and reducing the amount of surgery needed.

How Famotidine Works

Famotidine acts by reducing the amount of stomach acids secreted, as well as by reducing the output of pepsin. Its action is similar to that of cimetidine, in that it is a histamine H_2-receptor antagonist.

Recommended Dosage

The generally recommended dose is 40 milligrams daily by mouth at bedtime for four to eight weeks. Where appropriate, a maintenance dose of 20 milligrams daily may be given, also at bedtime.

Side Effects of Famotidine

Famotidine is readily absorbed by the gastric tract and should be used with caution by those with kidney disease or kidney failure. Generally, it is well tolerated, but adverse side effects may include diarrhea, dizziness, fatigue, and rashes. Unlike cimetidine, famotidine is reported to have little or no feminizing effect on men, and its potential for interacting with other drugs is also considered to be less.

Infrequently, confused states are experienced by people taking this medication, especially among the elderly or seriously ill. These are reversible; the person will regain normal orientation as soon as the drug is stopped. There have also been rare cases of allergic reactions, arthralgia, myalgia, blood disorders, nephritis, headache, hepatotoxicity, and pancreatitis.

FLUCLOXACILLIN

Flucloxacillin is a penicillin that is used primarily for the treatment of staphylococcal infections that are resistant to benzylpenicillin. This includes infections of the skin and soft tissues, bones and joints, respiratory and urinary tracts, middle ear, heart, blood, and brain. Flucloxacillin is also used to prevent staph infections during surgery.

How Flucloxacillin Works

Flucloxacillin is another synthetic penicillin, but it is absorbed by the gastrointestinal tract about twice as well as cloxacillin, so may be more suitable for certain types of infections. It is similar in action to benzylpenicillin but is stronger against some penicillin-resistant staph germs. It is less active against strep than benzylpenicillin.

Recommended Dosage

Flucloxacillin is taken in dosages of 250 milligrams four times daily. It can also be given by intramuscular injection. Dosages may be raised for severe infections. It should be taken before meals, as the presence of food in the stomach can reduce absorption. For children's dosages, your doctor should be consulted. This drug may be administered in conjunction with other antibiotics such as ampicillin, to give a broader spectrum of antibacterial activity.

Side Effects of Flucloxacillin

See cloxacillin.

FLUOCINOLONE ACETONIDE

Fluocinolone is a topical corticosteroid that is applied to the skin to treat a variety of skin disorders and conditions. It relieves itching, rash, or inflammation. It is available as a cream, gel, or ointment in concentrations ranging from .0025 to .2 percent.

How Fluocinolone Works

Fluocinolone is an anti-inflammatory that suppresses the manifestations of many conditions and is only one of many corticosteroids available to treat inflammations. The corticosteroids work by interfering with the body's mechanism of responding to an irritating or inflaming agent. Therefore, if the agent is not removed, i.e., the infection resolved, the corticosteroid will only suppress the symptoms.

Recommended Dosage

The strength of the preparation may vary. Apply in a thin film to clean skin.

Side Effects of Fluocinolone

There can be an increased vulnerability to fungal and viral infections if this product is used incorrectly. If treatment is prolonged, there may be side effects such as disturbances in bone marrow function. Other side effects include cessation of menstruation, mental or neurological disturbances, hairiness, bruising, and acne. There may also be loss of skin collagen and loss of skin pigmentation if this drug is overused.

Any corticosteroid carries the risk of being absorbed systemically (rather than just locally) if applied over large areas with great frequency. Once systemic, it can suppress the activity of the adrenal gland and cause electrolyte imbalance, metabolic disturbances, and retention of salt and water with resulting edema and high blood pressure. Infections which need treatment above and beyond the suppression of swelling or redness may actually be masked by this drug and worsen if left untreated.

FRUSEMIDE

Frusemide is a rapid-acting diuretic. Its effects are evident within thirty minutes to one hour after oral administration. It is used to treat edema, kidney insufficiency, or hypertension in situations where the thiazide family of diuretics don't work because higher dosages are required. (This is true because frusemide has a steep dose-response curve compared to the thiazides' flat dose-response curve.)

How Frusemide Works

Frusemide works by increasing the pace of urine production. It is a high ceiling diuretic because its strongest effect appears to be localized on the nephron's ascending limb.

Recommended Dosage

In treating edema, the usual initial dose is 40 milligrams once daily. Mild cases may respond to just 20 milligrams or 40 milligrams on alternate days. Some people may require 80 milligrams given as one or two daily doses. Children should be given this drug only at the suggestion and under the guidance of a physician.

Side Effects of Frusemide

The most common side effect associated with frusemide is electrolyte imbalance, particularly after large doses or a long period of time. This occurs when certain elements, such as potassium, are excreted in the urine in amounts large enough to interfere with the body's proper functioning.

Other side effects may include allergic reaction, nausea, diarrhea, blurred vision, dizziness, headache, sensitivity to light, and skin rashes; other conditions may occur rarely such as liver problems or pancreatitis. Ringing in the ears or even deafness have been known to occur. Frusemide may also cause attacks of gout or hyperglycemia.

Frusemide increases the amount of calcium that is excreted in the urine, and kidney stones have been reported.

FYBOGEL NATURAL HIGH FIBER REGIMEN*

This laxative contains ispaghula husk which is useful in the treatment of chronic constipation and when excessive straining at stool must be avoided, such as following surgery for hemorrhoids. Its ability to increase fecal mass also makes it useful in the treatment of diarrhea and for adjusting fecal consistency in patients with colostomies, diverticular disease, and irritable bowel syndrome.

How Fybogel Works

Ispaghula husk consists of the dried ripe seeds of the plantago plant. The husk swells rapidly in water, forming a stiff substance which provides intestinal bulk. It increases the fecal bulk and helps move the bowels by absorbing water in the intestinal tract.

Recommended Dosage

Ispaghula husk is administered in dosages of 3 to 5 milligrams, or one sachet, dissolved in water twice daily. The effect of bulk-forming laxatives is usually evident in twenty-four hours, but two to three days of medication may be necessary to achieve the desired effect.

Side Effects of Fybogel

Large quantities of ispaghula husk may temporarily increase flatulence and abdominal distension, and there is a risk of intestinal obstruction. Esophageal obstruction may occur if the substance is swallowed dry. Bulk laxatives also lower the transmission time through the colon, and so may affect the absorption of other drugs.

HEXAMINE HIPPURATE

Hexamine is used in the treatment of chronic recurrent, uncomplicated urinary tract infections primarily affecting the lower urinary tract, as well as in simple bacteriuria. It can also be used in prevention of those infections.

Hexamine is not suitable for upper urinary tract infections, because it is eliminated too rapidly to exert an effect. It is also not useful in acute infections, but rather in the chronic or recurring variety. Hexamine is recommended for long-term use because bacterial resistance does not seem to develop.

How Hexamine Works

The antibacterial action of hexamine is due to the formation of formaldehyde, which is created when hexamine is metabolized.

Recommended Dosage

The usual adult dose is 1 gram four times daily by mouth, after meals and at bedtime. Since it is only active in acid urine, it is important to take ammonium chloride or ascorbic acid at the same time. Some bacteria produce so much ammonia that the urine cannot be acidified and hexamine will not be effective.

Side Effects of Hexamine

Hexamine and its salts are usually well tolerated but may cause gastrointestinal disturbances such as nausea, vomiting, and diarrhea. The large amounts of formaldehyde that are by-products of its action may cause irritation and inflammation of the urinary tract, especially the bladder, and painful urination. Blood and protein may be found in the urine. There have been occasional skin rashes reported as well.

Hexamine and its salts should not be taken by people with impaired liver function, because ammonia is released into the gastrointestinal tract. Hexamine should also be avoided by people with impaired kidney function, severe dehydration, metabolic acidosis, or gout.

Using Hexamine in Combination with Other Drugs

Hexamine products should not be given at the same time as sulfa drugs, and substances that alkalize the urine such as acetazolamide or potassium citrate, should be avoided during hexamine therapy. Hexamine may interfere with laboratory tests for catecholamines, 17-hydroxycorticosteroids, and estrogens.

HYDROCORTISONE CREAM (1 PERCENT)

A popular anti-inflammatory, hydrocortisone may be used in the treatment of eczema, dermatitis resulting from allergic reaction to poison oak or poison ivy, minor sunburn, other skin inflammations and irritations, and in the treatment of psoriasis.

How Hydrocortisone Works

Hydrocortisone is a member of the family of adrenocorticosteroids, drugs which are synthesized from the adrenal gland. The adrenal gland helps regulate many of the body's functions, including fluid and electrolyte balance.

Steroids such as cortisone have been found to be useful in inhibiting the body's inflammatory response. This can be lifesaving, but steroids do not of themselves cure the underlying cause of the inflammation; they only suppress its outward appearance.

Recommended Dosage

Apply hydrocortisone cream sparingly to clean skin. The cream should be applied as often as directed and smoothed gently into the affected area. Hydrocortisone should not be applied to broken skin, nor should a bandage or dressing be placed over it. A bandage can increase absorption, and your system can absorb more of the drug than is indicated.

Side Effects of Hydrocortisone Cream

Occasional burning, itching, irritation, dryness, and various forms of dermatitis have been reported. In some cases, after prolonged use near the eyes, glaucoma and cataracts have occurred. Where there has been excessive application over a broad area of the body, systemic absorption has sometimes developed and produced reversible symptoms of Cushing's syndrome.

IMIPRAMINE HYDROCHLORIDE

Imipramine hydrochloride is a tricyclic antidepressant useful in treating a variety of problems. It can raise peoples' spirits, help with sleep disturbances, improve appetite, and give a feeling of more energy. If this drug is given to a depressed person, the person will experience an elevation of mood. Sedative or antianxiety effects may appear within a few days of treatment, but most antidepressant effects require several weeks of treatment.

Imipramine is used for agoraphobia, panic attacks, depression, childhood depression, eating disorders, obsessive-compulsive disorders, sexual disorders and dysfunctions, and certain sleep disorders such as narcolepsy and aggressive behavior during sleep. It has also been used to treat depressed people with heart disease and to help cardiac arrhythmias.

How Imipramine Hydrochloride Works

Tricyclic antidepressants have a complex action that is not fully understood, but they have been useful in relieving major depression and other psychological problems. The effect may have more to do with a dulling of depressive thoughts than with stimulating euphoria. Imipramine can induce sleep and may be prescribed for insomnia, although this is not its primary use.

Recommended Dosage

In the treatment of depression in adults, imipramine is given by mouth in doses of 25 milligrams, three times daily initially, gradually increasing to 50 milligrams, three or four times daily as necessary. Higher doses of up to 300 milligrams daily may be needed for the severely depressed or hospitalized patient. For adolescents and the elderly, a suggested dose is 10 milligrams at night, increasing to 25 milligrams three times daily.

Since imipramine has a long half-life and is slowly excreted, one dose, usually at bedtime is the preferred method. For treatment of bedwetting in children or childhood depression, consult your physician for guidance as to dosage. Two to three weeks may pass before the beneficial effects of this drug are apparent.

Side Effects of Imipramine Hydrochloride

Reactions to antidepressants are fairly common and include dry mouth, a sour or metallic taste in the mouth, stomach distress, constipation, dizziness, heart palpitations, blurred vision, excessive sweating, and urinary retention. Weakness and fatigue may also be experienced.

Another side effect of imipramine can be a switch from depressed to manic behavior. A tremor may also appear in some people. People with glaucoma must use this drug under the guidance of a physician. Some heart conditions, such as tachycardia and ventricular arrhythmias may be made worse by taking antidepressants. Also, the effect of other heart medication may be enhanced or otherwise affected.

Using Imipramine in Combination with Other Drugs

Imipramine may have reactions with other drugs including aspirin, phenytoin, aminopyrine, scopolamine, and phenothiazines. Cigarette smoking may increase the metabolism of antidepressants in the liver. People being treated with monoamine oxidase (MAO) inhibitors should never take this drug, as there is a chance of major reaction with high fevers, convulsions, or even death. Common MAO inhibitors are isoniazid, iproniazid, and phenelzine.

Imipramine enhances the effects of barbiturates, alcohol, and tranquilizers. Large doses of vitamin C or oral contraceptives can reduce the effects of imipramine. Bicarbonate of soda, acetazolamide, quinidine, and procainamide enhance the effect of imipramine and cause it to stay in the body longer, creating a potential for overdose.

ISOSORBIDE DINITRATE

Isosorbide dinitrate is used in the treatment of angina pectoris and other cardiac conditions, including congestive heart failure following a heart attack. It is also used for disorders of the esophagus and for certain types of hypertension.

How Isosorbide Dinitrate Works

Isosorbide is a vasodilator. That means it widens the blood vessels similarly to nitroglycerin and is used for many of the same purposes.

Recommended Dosage

Isosorbide can be swallowed or allowed to dissolve under the tongue. When a tablet is dissolved under the tongue, effects begin after about five minutes and last for about two hours. When swallowed, effects are evident after thirty minutes and last for up to five hours.

The usual dose for angina pectoris is 5 to 20 milligrams three times daily, according to the needs. Doses can be as high as 240 milligrams daily. Increases in dosages should be gradual in order to avoid side effects. For acute attacks of angina, the usual dose is 2.5 to 10 milligrams, under the tongue.

Like nitroglycerin, isosorbide is very volatile and may explode if subjected to excessive shaking or heat. This drug should be stored in a glass container and protected from heat and light.

Side Effects of Isosorbide Dinitrate

People with marked anemia or head injuries that may increase intracranial pressure should not use this drug. Isosorbide may increase pressure within the eye in people with glaucoma, and should be used with caution by people who have had liver or kidney problems. Prolonged contact with the skin may cause dermatitis, or tolerance and dependency leading to withdrawal symptoms. Some effects may be enhanced by alcohol.

ISOXSUPRINE HYDROCHLORIDE

Isoxsuprine is used in the treatment of cerebral and vascular disease. This medication has also been used to arrest premature labor. It provides relief of symptoms arising from chronic brain syndrome and assists in better memory and intellectual functions.

How Isoxsuprine Works

Isoxsuprine works by dilating the blood vessels and increasing the amount of blood supplied to the brain. It acts on the nerves that control the muscles in the major blood vessels and this, in theory, relaxes the muscles and allows more blood to flow to the brain.

Recommended Dosage

When used to increase brain functioning, the usual dose is 10 to 20 milligrams three to four times per day.

Side Effects of Isoxsuprine

Isoxsuprine may cause flushing and gastrointestinal disturbances. It may also cause birth defects or interfere with a baby's development. Other side effects include rapid heartbeat, nausea, vomiting, dizziness, stomach distress, and severe rash.

Another side effect of isoxsuprine is low blood pressure. This can result in light-headedness or dizziness. If you are taking this or any other vasodilator, be sure not to stand for long periods of time and do not get out of bed or stand up too quickly.

LATAMOXEF DISODIUM

Latamoxef disodium is a cephalosporin-based antibiotic, similar to third-generation cephalosporins. It is active against a wide range of bacteria, including many gram-positive and gram-negative organisms, genital tract infections and gastrointestinal infections. It is sometimes used in combination with other antibiotics such as penicillins for greater impact.

How Latamoxef Disodium Works

Latamoxef disodium works like other members of the cephalosporin family by inhibiting bacterial cell-wall synthesis.

Recommended Dosage

The usual dosage for adults is .5 to 4 grams daily, in two divided doses. For serious infections, this may be increased to up to 4 grams every eight hours. However at these levels, there may be a risk of bleeding disorders, and vitamin K may be prescribed by the physician to accompany the therapy. Infants and children may be given doses of 50 milligrams per kilogram of body weight every twelve hours; those aged one to four weeks, 25 milligrams per kilogram every eight hours. Those doses may be doubled in serious infections.

Side Effects of Latamoxef Disodium

Latamoxef disodium should not be taken by people who are allergic to cephalosporins. Great care should also be used by people who are allergic to penicillin, as 10 percent of these may be sensitive to the cephalosporins as well. People with kidney impairment or people who are taking diuretic medications should use this drug with caution. Kidney function and blood status must be monitored during long-term and high-dose therapy.

Allergic reactions to this medication have included skin rashes, fevers, anaphylaxis, and anemia. Prolonged use may result in overgrowth of resistant organisms and colitis. There is also a possibility of aggravating bleeding disorders. Blood coagulation time may be impaired by this drug, and aspirin or other nonsteroidal anti-inflammatory drugs may increase the risk of bleeding.

LINCOMYCIN HYDROCHLORIDE

Lincomycin hydrochloride, an antibiotic, was named because it was originally refined from the soil near Lincoln, Nebraska. It is prescribed for serious anaerobic bacterial infections, including some protozoal infections, and is recommended as an alternative to penicillin in some staph and strep infections, including staph infections of the bone. Because it does not penetrate the blood-brain barrier, it is not used to treat infections of the central nervous system.

How Lincomycin Hydrochloride Works

Lincomycin hydrochloride distributes itself widely throughout the tissues of the body and is excreted in the milk of nursing mothers. Its relative, clindamycin, is usually preferred because of its better absorption and fewer side effects.

Recommended Dosage

Lincomycin hydrochloride is administered by mouth in 500 milligram dosages three to four times daily, taken at least one hour before eating. Higher doses may be given in very severe infections. Children over age one month may be given 30 to 60 milligrams per kilogram of body weight daily in divided doses by mouth.

Side Effects of Lincomycin Hydrochloride

Lincomycin hydrochloride should not be taken by people who are known to be hypersensitive to it or who have experienced reactions to clindamycin. Kaolin and cyclamates reduce the absorption of lincomycin hydrochloride from the gastrointestinal tract. This drug may cause diarrhea, persistent nausea and vomiting, severe colitis, skin rashes, urticaria, leukopenia, eosinophilia, and liver jaundice.

LOPERAMIDE HYDROCHLORIDE

Loperamide hydrochloride is used for the control of acute and chronic diarrhea and diarrhea associated with inflammatory bowel disease.

How Loperamide Hydrochloride Works

Loperamide hydrochloride acts by slowing the activity (motility) of the intestine, as well as by slowing the passage of water through the bowel. It also inhibits the peristaltic action of the intestines by its effect on the muscles of the intestinal wall.

Recommended Dosage

The recommended initial dose is two capsules (2 milligrams each) or four teaspoonsful of liquid (4 milligrams) followed by one capsule or two teaspoonfuls of liquid (2 milligrams) after each unformed stool. Daily dosage should not exceed eight capsules or sixteen teaspoonfuls of liquid (16 milligrams). Improvement should be noticed within forty-eight hours.

Loperamide hydrochloride is not recommended for use in children under two years of age. In older children it should be taken following your physician's guidance.

Side Effects of Loperamide Hydrochloride

Adverse reactions include skin rashes, abdominal pain, nausea and vomiting, constipation, tiredness, drowsiness or dizziness, and dry mouth. Loperamide hydrochloride should not be used in cases of acute dysentery or if abdominal distention occurs, and should be used with caution by patients with liver disease. People with liver disease should be carefully monitored by their physician when taking this drug.

METFORMIN HYDROCHLORIDE

Metformin hydrochloride is used to treat non–insulin-dependent diabetes when diet control fails. It is combined with insulin in the treatment of insulin-dependent diabetes. It is also recommended when other diabetic drugs, such as the sulfonylureas of chlorpropamides have failed to work, or become ineffective. Metformin hydrochloride is sometimes given to overweight people to help them lose weight.

How Metformin Hydrochloride Works

Metformin hydrochloride seems to work by causing a person to develop a mild form of hypoglycemia, thus lowering their blood sugar. It does not stimulate insulin release but requires that some insulin be present in order for it to work.

Recommended Dosage

Metformin hydrochloride is given by mouth initially at 500 milligrams three times per day, or 850 milligrams twice daily with meals, and gradually increased, if necessary, to a maximum of 3 grams daily.

Side Effects of Metformin Hydrochloride

Metformin hydrochloride has been a controversial drug, which can cause adverse side effects, such as loss of appetite, nausea, and vomiting. The body's ability to absorb vitamin B12 and other substances may be impaired by it. Other side effects include a metallic taste, weight loss, and an increase in blood lipid concentrations.

A serious, sometimes fatal condition called lactic acidosis has been reported, but to a lesser extent than with the related drug phenformin. It has generally occurred only in people whose medical condition indicated that they should not have begun metformin hydrochloride therapy.

Metformin hydrochloride should not be used by people who have had heart failure, dehydration, acute or chronic alcoholism, or any other condition that may cause a possibility of lactic acidosis. People with kidney impairment should take this drug only on the advice of their physician.

METRONIDAZOLE HYDROCHLORIDE

Metronidazole hydrochloride is used in the treatment of vaginal infections such as trichomoniasis and other anaerobic protozoal and bacterial infections. It is also used in treating amebic dysentery and other parasitic diseases. It may be prescribed even when there are no symptoms of infection, if testing shows that there are bacteria or protozoa present.

When this drug is used to treat trichomonal vaginal infections, the partner should also be treated since reinfection is possible and this infection can also be passed on.

How Metronidazole Hydrochloride Works

Metronidazole hydrochloride is believed to work by interfering with the DNA of the microorganism that is causing the infection. Resistance to metronidazole hydrochloride seems to be rare. Because it is rapidly absorbed, it should be supplemented with other drugs when treating amebic dysentery.

Recommended Dosage

Metronidazole hydrochloride is given by mouth in tablets, in oral suspension. It can also be given rectally, by suppositories. The tablets are taken with or after food, and the suspension at least one hour before food. The frequency of dosage should be reduced for people with liver disease, and possibly in newborns or the elderly. The dosage may vary, depending upon the type of infection being treated, so consult your doctor before starting a course of metronidazole hydrochloride.

Side Effects of Metronidazole Hydrochloride

The adverse effects of metronidazole hydrochloride are often dose related. The most common side effects are gastrointestinal disturbance and nausea, an unpleasant metallic taste, headache, loss of appetite, vomiting, diarrhea, dry mouth, a furred tongue, glossitis, and stomatitis. Rarely, a case of colitis may develop. Some people have experienced numbness and tingling in the arms and legs, and extremely high doses or extended treatment have caused seizures in sensitive people. Weakness, dizziness and disorientation, drowsiness, changes in mood, depression, and confusion have been reported.

Metronidazole hydrochloride may cause birth defects, so pregnant women should not use it unless recommended by a physician. Metronidazole hydrochloride should not be used by women who are breast-feeding their babies, as it is passed through the breast milk. It has also been shown to be carcinogenic (cancer causing) in animals, but the effects on man are not at present fully known.

People who have a disease of the nervous system should use this product with care, as should people with blood dyscrasias. People taking metronidazole hydrochloride may develop moderate leukopenia, skin rashes, and pruritus. Thrombophlebitis has occasionally followed intravenous injection, as have elevated liver enzymes.

Using Metronidazole Hydrochloride in Combination with Other Drugs

When metronidazole hydrochloride is taken with alcohol, some people have become extremely ill. It should not be taken with disulfiram, as it has caused acute psychoses and confusion. Phenobarbitone may diminish the effectiveness of metronidazole hydrochloride. Cimetidine has been known to increase the blood concentrations of metronidazole hydrochloride and thus could increase the possibility of neurological side effects. Because of its action, metronidazole hydrochloride may mask some symptoms of early syphilis.

MICONAZOLE NITRATE

Miconazole nitrate is an antifungal agent that is also active against several strains of staph and strep infections. It has been used to treat candidiasis, coccidioidomycosis and other strains of infection, such as ringworm, pityriasis versicolor, and acne, as well as fungal meningitis. It has also been used as a preventive by people who are at high risk of opportunistic fungal infections. In lower concentrations, it is effective against common fungus infections such as jock itch and athlete's foot.

How Miconazole Nitrate Works

Miconazole nitrate works by penetrating the stratum corneum of the skin and causing it to shed its surface cells. The fungus inhabits the stratum corneum and is removed in the process.

Recommended Dosage

Miconazole nitrate may be applied to the skin, taken orally, or injected in the dosages prescribed by your doctor.

Side Effects of Miconazole Nitrate

Following injection of miconazole nitrate, people have experienced vein irritation, itching, rash, nausea, vomiting, fever, drowsiness, diarrhea, loss of appetite, and flushing; some people have reported rapid or irregular heartbeat. There may be itching or burning after vaginal administration, pelvic cramps, hives, rash, headache; skin irritation or burning may follow topical application.

MINOXIDIL

Minoxidil is prescribed for high blood pressure that is not controllable with other drugs. When used to treat high blood pressure, minoxidil is usually given in combination with other drugs such as beta blockers as part of an overall program of therapy. In topical form, it is also used as a 1 to 5 percent lotion to treat male baldness.

How Minoxidil Works

Minoxidil works by dilating the blood vessels, thus causing a drop in blood pressure. More blood then flows through the arms and legs. This reduces the amount of work that the heart has to accomplish to pump blood through the body.

It is not fully understood why minoxidil stimulates the growth of hair in some men, but it may act by stimulating the hair follicle. The response rate varies according to the degree of baldness and concentration of the ointment. Men who have been bald for a shorter duration of time and who have not lost a great amount of hair seem to respond the best.

Recommended Dosage

Dosages vary, and there is still debate as to the best concentration. A 2 percent lotion has shown good response when applied twice daily for up to six months. The treatment must be continued in order for the hair growth to be maintained. When using minoxidil to manage high blood pressure, consult a physician for the appropriate dosage.

Side Effects of Minoxidil

Adverse effects of oral minoxidil may include a rapid heartbeat, fluid retention, weight gain, edema, and sometimes congestive heart failure. This is why it is usually given with a beta blocker and diuretic. Minoxidil may uncover or aggravate angina pectoris. Other side effects may include breast growth in men, nausea, allergic skin rashes, polymenorrhea, and thrombocytopenia.

Minoxidil should be discontinued if pulse increases twenty or more beats per minute, if there is difficulty in breathing, faintness, chest pain, dizziness, or unusual swelling.

NEOMYCIN SULFATE WITH BACITRACIN

Neomycin is an antibiotic similar to gentamicin, which is active against many strains of bacteria. Bacitracin is another antibiotic which is added to help prevent the emergence of resistant strains of the germs. Neomycin is used for topical infections of the skin and eye, especially those caused by staphylococci or other sensitive organisms.

How Neomycin Sulfate with Bacitracin Works

Neomycin sulfate works by preventing the growth of bacteria through the inhibition of protein synthesis. Bacitracin works by interfering with the synthesis of the cell walls of bacteria.

Recommended Dosage

Follow your physician's directions and apply to the affected area no more often than advised. Do not take this preparation internally.

Side Effects of Neomycin Sulfate with Bacitracin

Frequent or long-term use of this medication may lead to the development of strains of bacteria resistant to the ointment. This drug can be absorbed systemically. When applied as an aerosol to open wounds or damaged skin, neomycin can enter the system and cause partial or total irreversible deafness, especially in cases where there is liver or kidney impairment. Neomycin has an intramuscular blocking action that may also cause breathing difficulty or arrest.

NIFEDIPINE

Nifedipine is used in the treatment of angina pectoris, especially where there is spasm of the blood vessels, in treating hypertension, and in Raynaud's phenomenon, as well as for the treatment of asthma.

How Nifedipine Works

Nifedipine is a calcium channel blocker, which works primarily to dilate coronary and peripheral arteries and reduce blood pressure. It increases heart rate, coronary blood flow, oxygen supply, and overall coronary output.

Recommended Dosage

The usual oral dose is 10 milligrams three times daily, taken during or after meals, increased to 20 milligrams if necessary three times daily. A maximum daily dose of 180 milligrams has been suggested. A recommended initial dose for elderly patients is 5 milligrams three times daily.

Side Effects of Nifedipine

Nifedipine should be used with caution by people who have hypotension or whose cardiac output is poor. The use of nifedipine in diabetic patients may require adjustment of diabetic treatment. It should be discontinued in people who suffer ischemic pain following its administration. Possible adverse reactions include dizziness, flushing, headache, hypotension, and peripheral edema.

NITROFURANTOIN

Nitrofurantoin is active against several bacteria, including *Escherichia coli*, enterococci, *Staphylococcus aureus*, and *Staphylococcus epidermis*. It is useful in urinary tract infections because it appears in great concentrations in the urine. Because it does not concentrate in the blood, it is not useful for other types of infections. Nitrofurantoin is used to control infections of the urinary tract, including urethral infractions, bladder infections, pyelonephritis, and pyelitis. It is used to prevent and to treat long-term infections.

How Nitrofurantoin Works

Nitrofurantoin acts by interfering with the enzyme systems of the affected bacteria.

Recommended Dosage

Nitrofurantoin is best taken with food to improve drug absorption and tolerance. Adult dose is usually 50 to 100 milligrams four times a day. For uncomplicated urinary tract infections a lowered dosage is usually sufficient. Children receive 5 to 7 milligrams per kilogram of body weight every twenty-four hours in four divided doses. Nitrofurantoin is continued for at least three days after urine becomes sterile. If no improvement is noted within that time, therapy must be reevaluated since the bacteria may be resistant to this drug.

Side Effects of Nitrofurantoin

Nitrofurantoin is not for use by infants or pregnant women. Occasional side effects include nausea, vomiting, abdominal pain, diarrhea, headache, drowsiness, and allergic reactions such as skin rash.

OXYTETRACYCLINE

Tetracycline was developed as a result of a worldwide effort to collect soil specimens for their antibiotic-producing organisms. The first tetracycline was introduced in 1948 and oxytetracycline came into being two years later. The tetracyclines soon become widely used in antibacterial therapy as they act against both gram-positive and gram-negative bacteria.

The tetracyclines are useful in treating a wide variety of infections including typhus; Rocky Mountain spotted fever; Q fever; chlamydia, trachoma, and other eye infections; brucellosis; bubonic plague, venereal diseases, chronic bronchitis, syphilis, urinary tract infections, acne, tropical sprue, Whipple's disease, cholera, Lyme disease, leptospirosis, malaria, amebic dysentery, yaws, and gingivitis.

How Oxytetracycline Works

Once the drug makes its way into the bacterial cell, it interferes with the function of the cell and destroys it.

Many bacteria have developed resistance to tetracyclines. The incidence of these problems seems to be higher with the tetracyclines than with the penicillins. Because of the resistance of certain strains of staph, strep, or meningococcal bacteria, tetracyclines are not generally used for these types of infections.

Recommended Dosage

Oxytetracycline is best taken on an empty stomach with an eight-ounce glass of water, one or two hours after a meal. Sometimes dairy products such as milk or cheese may interfere with the effect of this drug. The usual adult dosage is 250 to 500 milligrams four times per day. For children nine years old or over, 50 to 100 milligrams four times per day. A child under age eight should not take this drug since it may lead to discolored adult teeth.

Side Effects of Oxytetracycline

Various skin rashes and dermatitis may follow the use of oxytetracycline, but these are rare. However, allergic reactions and even anaphylactic reactions have been known to occur after oral use of tetracyclines. People who have a history of allergies, or who are sensitive to any of the tetracyclines, should not use this drug. Unused tetracycline should always be discarded since it can break down into a dangerous form after the expiration date.

Treatment of pregnant women by tetracyclines has been shown to discolor the teeth of the unborn child. Tetracyclines may also interfere with bone growth of the fetus when taken by pregnant women. The most common side effects of tetracyclines are irritated stomach, nausea, vomiting, and diarrhea. Irritated esophagus has also been reported, usually due to an insufficient amount of water being taken with the pill. Fatty changes in the liver and pancreatitis have been reported in pregnant women taking tetracyclines intravenously for kidney infections or in those with kidney impairment.

Suprainfections such as candida, vaginitis, and diarrhea have occurred with strains resistant to tetracyclines after long-time use. People with kidney impairment should take this drug with caution and under the advice of a physician.

Using Oxytetracycline in Combination with Other Drugs

Tetracyclines should not be taken with drugs that may affect the liver, such as erythromycin, estolate, chloramphenicol, sulfa drugs, aminosalicylic acid, isoniazid, chlorpromazine phenytoin, and chlorpropamide. Tetracyclines may enhance the effects of oral anticoagulants and diminish the effectiveness of oral contraceptives. Vitamin and mineral supplements can reduce the effectiveness of tetracyclines.

PANCORIN*

Pancorin is actually nitroglycerin that is dispensed from a skin patch. Nitroglycerin is useful against the pain of angina pectoris, pulmonary hypertension, and in relieving spasms of the esophagus. It is sometimes used in alleviating the effects of ongoing heart attacks.

How Pancorin Works

Nitroglycerin works by relaxing smooth muscle, including vascular muscle, and reducing the blood pressure. It limits the heart's demand for oxygen by dilating the vessels of the heart and decreasing arterial resistance. This medication is absorbed rapidly through the mucosal lining, which is why tablets are often dissolved under the tongue.

Recommended Dosage

Administration of nitroglycerin via transdermal patches has several advantages including convenience, accuracy of dosage, and patient acceptance. Some believe that tolerance is more likely to develop as a consequence of steady administration via patch than with intermittent sublingual dosage. For this reason, it has been suggested that the patch be worn eight to sixteen hours per day.

Side Effects of Pancorin

This drug should not be used by people with marked anemia or with raised intracranial pressure due to head trauma or cerebral hemorrhage. People with glaucoma, constrictive pericarditis, severe hypotension, or impaired kidney or liver function should use this drug with caution. Side effects that have been reported include flushing, dizziness, tachycardia, and headache. Vomiting, restlessness, hypotension, and coldness of the skin have also been occasionally reported.

PENICILLIN V POTASSIUM

Penicillin V potassium is useful only in the treatment of mild to moderate infections and is not suitable for chronic or severe infections. This medication is often used before dental work to prevent infection, as well as for the treatment of Lyme disease, anthrax, strep infections, tonsillitis, and to prevent recurrent attacks of rheumatic fever and Whipple's disease.

Penicillin V potassium is resistant to being neutralized

by stomach acids, so it is suitable to take by mouth. Its calcium and potassium salts aid in absorption.

How Penicillin V Potassium Works

Penicillin V potassium works like the rest of the penicillin family by breaking down the cell wall and, consequently, killing susceptible bacteria.

Recommended Dosage

The usual dosage for adults is 125 to 500 milligrams every four to six hours and is best taken on an empty stomach, thirty minutes before or two hours after eating. Consult your doctor for children's dosages. Dosage may need to be modified if there is severe kidney impairment. This antibiotic should be taken in an upright position with at least eight ounces of water to prevent ulcers of the esophagus. Be sure to take all the penicillin recommended in order to clear up the infection, and store this drug in the refrigerator.

Side Effects of Penicillin V Potassium

Penicillin V potassium is generally well tolerated but may cause nausea and diarrhea. Adverse effects are similar to those of benzylpenicillin, namely skin rashes, and risk of anaphylactic shock and death has been reported. Urticaria, fever, joint pains, hemolitic anemia, leukopenia, lengthening of bleeding time, and changes in blood have also been reported. Very high doses may cause convulsions, particularly in people with impaired kidneys. Sometimes fever and chills can be the result of toxins released by the dying bacteria. A sore mouth or black, hairy tongue may also occur.

Using Penicillin V Potassium in Combination with Other Drugs

The drug probenecid lengthens the time it takes to excrete penicillin from the body. Some nonsteroidal anti-inflammatory drugs compete with penicillin for room in the kidneys. Penicillin may interfere with some diagnostic tests, such as urinary glucose and some tests for urinary or serum proteins. People who have bone marrow failure need to be medicated with special care because of the risk of suprainfection. Penicillin V potassium should not be taken if you are using erythromycin, tetracycline, or neomycin, as they may interfere with the penicillin.

PHENYLBUTAZONE

Phenylbutazone is used to help relieve the pain of arthritis, gout, rheumatoid arthritis, ankylosing spondylitis, osteoarthritis, bursitis, inflammation of a joint, or other conditions where milder drugs such as aspirin have proven ineffective. It should only be used after nonsteroidal anti-inflammatory therapy has been tried first. Phenylbutazone is for symptomatic relief of rheumatoid problems and does nothing to alter the disease process.

How Phenylbutazone Works

Phenylbutazone works like the rest of the aspirin-like drugs. It inhibits the biosynthesis and release of prostaglandins in all cells.

Recommended Dosage

For adults and children over age fourteen, 300 to 600 milligrams per day in three or four equal doses for seven days. The high initial dose should be given for as short a time as possible and should be discontinued after a week if there is no improvement.

When improvement is noted, the dosage should be reduced to the smallest possible amount that will still be effective. Maintenance doses should not exceed 400 milligrams daily, and 100 to 200 milligrams may be adequate. Blood counts should be taken frequently during the course of treatment, and the medication should be stopped completely if there are any reactions or symptoms of toxicity.

Side Effects of Phenylbutazone

Phenylbutazone can cause gastric or duodenal ulcer, perforation of the large bowel, bleeding from the stomach, anemia, vomiting, nausea, diarrhea, vomiting of blood, hepatitis which can be fatal, kidney bleeding, and kidney stones. You should not take this drug if you have ever had stomach problems, such as an ulcer, or any gastrointestinal inflammation. Phenylbutazone has been known to cause inflammation of the heart and damage to bone marrow. Sometimes this damage to the bone marrow may arise suddenly.

PIRENZEPINE HYDROCHLORIDE

Pirenzepine hydrochloride is used in the treatment of duodenal, peptic, and gastric ulcers. It is absorbed by the gastrointestinal tract, and the efficiency of absorption is decreased from 25 percent to 10 to 20 percent when the medication is taken with food. The ulcer healing which takes place with pirenzepine hydrochloride is thought to be dose-related. Doses of 100 to 150 milligrams improved the healing rates of peptic ulcers significantly, a rate comparable with that of cimetidine. However, it has been shown to act more slowly than cimetidine.

How Pirenzepine Hydrochloride Works

Pirenzepine hydrochloride acts by binding chemically to the receptors of the gastric mucosa and causing a reduction in the secretion of gastric acid, as well as in the production of pepsin.

Recommended Dosage

The usual dose is 50 milligrams twice daily by mouth for four to six weeks. If necessary, the dosage may be increased to 50 milligrams three times daily. Pirenzepine hydrochloride may be administered for up to three months under the direction of a physician, and should be taken on an empty stomach before meals for optimum effect. It can also be taken in a low dosage (30 to 50 milligrams daily) in long-term therapy to help prevent ulcer recurrence.

Side Effects of Pirenzepine Hydrochloride

Adverse reactions may include dry mouth and blurred vision, diarrhea, constipation, headache, and mental confusion. Because pirenzepine hydrochloride penetrates the blood-brain barrier poorly, there are fewer psychological side effects associated with it.

PREDNISOLONE/PREDNISONE

Prednisolone is classified as an anti-inflammatory drug. It is the medication of choice whenever corticosteroid therapy is necessary. It is used to treat skin rashes, diseases, insufficiency of the adrenal gland, arthritis and bursitis, skin rashes ranging from psoriasis to poison ivy, serum sickness, conjunctivitis, blood disorders, diseases of the stomach and large intestine, ulcerative colitis, and many inflammations. Corticosteroids are also used in cancer treatment to minimize the aftereffects of chemotherapy.

Unlike prednisone, prednisolone is already active and does not need to be converted into active form by the liver. So for people with liver impairment, prednisolone is usually preferable to prednisone. Application of these preparations to the skin often results in dramatic improvement in many diseases such as eczema, dermatitis, some forms of psoriasis, although psoriasis may get worse after the drug is withdrawn.

How Prednisolone Works

The corticosteroids suppress the body's immune reactions and also the manifestations of many diseases. They do not correct the underlying cause of the disease, but only mask its symptoms. Since the body produces corticosteroids naturally in the adrenal gland, taking prednisolone can also suppress the action of the adrenal gland.

Recommended Dosage

The initial dose is 5 to 60 or more milligrams, with maintenance doses depending upon the purpose of the treatment. The lowest effective dose is generally the best course.

During periods of stress, following surgery, or during infections the dosage may need to be increased. Treatment may be intermittent, allowing the body to regain its metabolic balance, so two days' dose or a dose on alternate days is often used. People taking prednisolone should not be vaccinated against any diseases, since the body cannot react normally to the vaccine. Pregnant or nursing women should not take this medication.

131

Side Effects of Prednisolone

Side effects of prednisolone include stomach upset, gastric or duodenal ulcers, water retention, heart failure, muscle weakness or loss of muscle, loss of calcium, bone degeneration, black and blue marks, slower healing of wounds, sweating, allergic skin reactions such as rashes, convulsions, headache, or dizziness. Many abnormal effects are due to excessive use or overdosage. Growth retardation in children has been reported, as well as inflammation of the pancreas, moon face, hairiness, buffalo hump, acne, and sometimes Cushing's syndrome. Most of these side effects go away when the drug is stopped.

Oral administration of steroids can cause ulcers, diabetes, fluid pressure in the eyes, blood clots, a feeling of malaise or sickness, and psychological abnormalities such as mood swings, personality changes, and depression. If these conditions already exist, prednisolone may make them worse.

PROMETHAZINE HYDROCHLORIDE

Promethazine hydrochloride is an antihistamine used to treat coughs and colds, motion sickness, allergic reactions, and certain minor pains. Sometimes it is used as a light sedative, as well.

How Promethazine Works

The drug diminishes the actions of histamines in the body. Since antihistamines alleviate allergic manifestations, they are used for relief of itching and sneezing due to hay fever, mild allergic reactions to blood transfusions, serum sickness, and as a hypnotic to induce sleep or sedate a person prior to surgery. The effects of promethazine hydrochloride last from six to twelve hours.

Recommended Dosage

Promethazine hydrochloride is usually given at night in doses of 25 milligrams for allergic conditions, because of its sedative effect. Up to 60 milligrams per day may be administered in divided doses. This drug has not been established as safe for use in pregnancy, and it is not intended for children, unless directed by a physician.

Side Effects of Promethazine

Reported reactions include drowsiness, dizziness, listlessness, ringing in the ears, loss of coordination, fatigue, blurred vision, euphoria, double vision, nervousness, insomnia, tremors, convulsions, catatonia, and hysteria. Some users have experienced rapid or slowed heartbeat, faintness, and increases or decreases in blood pressure.

Promethazine hydrochloride may impair the alertness needed for driving or operating machinery, so it should not be used with sedatives, tranquilizers, or alcohol. This drug may significantly affect the action of other drugs, especially other depressants.

People who are asthmatic, who have glaucoma, prostatic hypertrophy, peptic ulcer, intestinal obstruction, pyloroduodenal obstruction, or bladder obstruction should use this drug with caution, under the guidance of a physician. Promethazine hydrochloride should also be used with caution if you have bone marrow depression, or either liver or kidney impairment.

PROPRANOLOL HYDROCHLORIDE

Propranolol hydrochloride is a beta blocker, prescribed to treat such conditions as high blood pressure, heart arrhythmias and irregularities, and heart attack, to prevent migraine headaches, and to treat tremors of the upper limbs which are not caused by Parkinson's disease.

Propranolol hydrochloride helps improve the tolerance to exercise for people with angina pectoris. It has been used to help people with stage fright and other anxiety reactions, as well. Propranolol hydrochloride is useful in treating certain types of heart arrhythmias, such as tachycardia or rapid heartbeat. There is evidence that propranolol hydrochloride reduces the chances of a second heart attack.

How Propranolol Hydrochloride Works

Propranolol hydrochloride works by reducing the activity of the heart. By blocking the reception of a natural body chemical that stimulates the heart, propranolol hydrochloride reduces the rate and force of contraction of the heart and decreases the rate at which stimulating impulses are conducted through the body. Its main effect is to reduce the response of the heart to stress—either emotional or physical—and to reduce blood pressure.

Recommended Dosage

The dosage of propranolol hydrochloride depends on the condition that is being treated. To treat high blood pressure the usual beginning dose is 40 milligrams twice daily, which may be increased gradually to 120 to 240 milligrams per day or higher. The time needed to calculate response may vary from days to several weeks. For prevention of migraines, the dose is 80 milligrams daily in divided doses. The usual effective dose range is 160 to 240 milligrams per day. To treat essential tremor, the usual dose is 40 milligrams twice daily. Optimum reduction of tremor is usually achieved with a dose of 120 milligrams per day.

Side Effects of Propranolol Hydrochloride

People have occasionally experienced the following side effects: decrease of heart rate; aggravation of congestive heart failure; lowered blood pressure; tingling in the fingers, arms, and legs; light-headedness; mental depression; inability to sleep; tiredness; and weakness. Others have reported hallucinations, visual disturbances, disorientation, short-term memory loss, nausea, vomiting, stomach upset, abdominal cramps, diarrhea, and constipation. Allergic reactions may include sore throat, fever, difficulty in breathing, and bronchospasms. There may be personality changes in some people or a feeling of detachment.

Propranolol should be used carefully if you have a history of upper respiratory disease such as bronchitis or asthma, or allergies. This drug may make these conditions worse. This medication should be used with caution if you have diabetes. You should not take propranolol if you have congestive heart failure, cardiogenic shock, slow heartbeat, or bronchial asthma. It is important that this drug not be discontinued abruptly, because there have been reports of worsening angina or even heart attacks if therapy is stopped suddenly.

Using Propranolol Hydrochloride in Combination with Other Drugs

Propranolol may interact with certain drugs such as reserpine, verapamil, or MAO inhibitors. It may also increase the effect of insulin or oral diabetic drugs. Propranolol may reduce the effectiveness of digitalis on your heart. Aluminum hydroxide gel and alcoholic beverages will reduce the absorption of propranolol, while drugs such as phenytoin, phenobarbitone and rifampin will speed absorption.

RANITIDINE

Ranitidine assists in the treatment of gastric and duodenal ulcers and other conditions that are helped by the suppression of stomach acid.

How Ranitidine Works

Ranitidine is of the same family of drugs as cimetidine, namely histamine H_2-receptor antagonists, which means they inhibit the production of stomach acid. Ranitidine is thoroughly absorbed when taken by mouth and causes immediate reduction of the secretion of acid. Over a twenty-four-hour period, there is up to a 50 percent reduction.

Recommended Dosage

The usual oral dose is 150 milligrams twice daily, once in the morning and once at bedtime. A single bedtime dose of 300 milligrams may be substituted in the management of duodenal and gastric ulcers. Treatment should initially be continued for at least four weeks. If appropriate, a maintenance dose may be given at bedtime of 150 milligrams daily. People with impaired kidney functions require a reduced dose.

Side Effects of Ranitidine

Considering the large number of people who have taken these drugs, the adverse side effects are relatively infrequent and generally minor. The most commonly reported side effects are headache, dizziness, diarrhea, constipation, and skin rashes. Unlike cimetidine, ranitidine does not have the side effects of impotence or gynecomastia. The potential for drug interactions is also considered less with ranitidine than with cimetidine.

RESERPINE

Reserpine is used to decrease high blood pressure in people who have not responded to a diuretic or beta blocker alone. It has also been used as a sedative in anxious people. Reserpine was formerly used to treat psychoses, but there are now many more effective drugs available for that purpose.

How Reserpine Works

Reserpine is obtained from the roots of certain species of rauwolfia plants. Rauwolfia drugs may take some time to become effective and have a sustained action that continues even after a person stops taking the drug.

Recommended Dosage

The recommended daily dose is 250 to 500 milligrams for the first two weeks. Thereafter, the dose should be reduced to the lowest possible level that maintains the decrease in blood pressure.

Side Effects of Reserpine

Side effects may include nasal congestion, depression, drowsiness, lethargy, nightmares, diarrhea, abdominal cramps, and excess secretion of gastric acid. Difficulty in breathing, anorexia, cyanosis, and hypothermia have occurred in infants whose mothers took reserpine before delivery. Breast enlargement, decreased sex drive, impotence, sodium retention, edema, increased appetite, and weight gain have also been reported.

This drug should not be taken by people who are mentally depressed or have suicidal tendencies. Reserpine may also impair the faculties needed for driving or operating machinery. It should not be taken by people who have a history of peptic ulcer, ulcerative colitis, or by people receiving electroshock therapy.

RETINOIC ACID

Retinoic acid is used to treat acne vulgaris and its comedones, papules, and pustules. It has also been used in the treatment of psoriasis and other skin disorders and recently, for the treatment of aging and skin damage and wrinkling caused by sun. It has been mentioned as a treatment for certain types of skin cancer as well.

How Retinoic Acid Works

Retinoic acid is actually a vitamin A preparation that acts by increasing the speed of the life processes of skin cells, allowing them to be sloughed off sooner. Thus the formation of whiteheads and other acne lesions is suppressed and the skin becomes clearer.

Recommended Dosage

The skin should be washed with soap and water prior to using retinoic acid and dried fifteen to twenty minutes before applying retinoic acid lightly, once or twice daily. Retinoic acid may cause stinging and a feeling of warmth. Do not apply retinoic acid to the eyes, mucous membranes, mouth, or nose. Use caution when using with other skin creams.

Side Effects of Retinoic Acid

People just beginning to use retinoic acid may notice at first that the acne appears to be worse, but this condition rapidly resolves with continued treatment. Most people should not stop using this if the pustules and acne appear to be growing worse, as that is part of the treatment process.

Allergic contact dermatitis and changes in skin color may necessitate a visit to the dermatologist. Blistering, crusting, and severe burning of the skin and irritation of the mucous membranes of the eyes, nose, and mouth may infrequently occur.

Retinoic acid sensitizes the skin to ultraviolet light and sunlight, so care should be taken to wear a sunblock or to limit exposure to the sun while using this preparation. People with eczema may be severely affected by the sun and should take extra precautions.

SODIUM PICOSULFATE

Sodium picosulfate is a laxative used to treat constipation and to assist in emptying the bowel before surgery. Its action takes place generally in the large intestine, and it is usually effective within ten to fourteen hours; however, when combined with magnesium citrate, it may work in just three hours.

How Sodium Picosulfate Works

Sodium picosulfate works by stimulating intestinal movement and increasing the amount of water and electrolytes in the bowels.

Recommended Dosage

Sodium picosulfate is given in doses for adults of 5 to 15 milligrams, usually at bedtime. Doses of 2.5 milligrams are recommended for children up to five years of age, and doses of 2.5 to 5 milligrams for children five to ten years of age.

Side Effects of Sodium Picosulfate

Sodium picosulfate may cause stomach discomfort such as colic. Prolonged use or overdose can cause diarrhea with resultant loss of electrolytes such as potassium and water. There is also a possibility of loss of flexibility in the colon.

This product should not be given to people with an intestinal obstruction or with undiagnosed stomach pain or other symptoms, or to people with inflammatory bowel disease. Children with undiagnosed stomach pain may have appendicitis or another condition. They should not be given laxatives except on the advice and under the guidance of a physician.

SULFA DRUGS (SULFADIAZINE, SULFAGUANADINE, SULFADIMIDINE, SULFATHIAZOLE, SULFASALAZINE)

These drugs all belong to the family of sulfanilamides, which were among the first drugs used to prevent and cure infections in man. Before penicillin became widely available, sulfanilamides were the mainstay of bacteriological therapy. By combining these drugs with other antibiotics, however, their effectiveness has been increased. Even though the sulfanilamides can kill bacteria in the body, the body's natural defenses are still necessary to completely eradicate the infection.

This family of drugs is used to treat infections, such as *E. coli*, and some staph and strep. They are also effective in preventing recurrences of rheumatic fever. The broad spectrum of infections that once was treated by these drugs has been diminished due to increased resistance of many strains of bacteria to them. Testing is often necessary to determine if the infection is treatable by any of these antibiotics.

How the Sulfa Drugs Work

The sulfa drugs work by preventing bacteria from completing their normal life functions and obtaining nutrients. Resistance occurs when the bacteria, which can mutate very rapidly, produce strains that do not respond to the drug and therefore survive, perpetuating the infection. Because the various sulfa drugs are absorbed differently, they are useful in treating different infections. Those that are absorbed very slowly are useful in treating bowel infections; those that act faster are used to treat urinary tract infections.

Recommended Dosage

The dosage may vary, depending upon your age, weight, medical condition, and the type of infection that is being treated. In people taking these types of drugs, it is always important to drink enough fluids.

Side Effects of the Sulfa Drugs

Nausea, vomiting, and diarrhea are fairly common side effects of the sulfa family of drugs. Other side effects may include rashes, light sensitivity, dermatitis, severe erythema multiforme with lesions over the body. There have been rare occurrences of back pain, blood in the urine, blood disorders, myocarditis, and pancreatitis.

Using Sulfa Drugs in Combination with Other Drugs

Taking sulfa drugs with certain other drugs such as anticoagulants may cause a release of larger amounts of these drugs than usual and produce symptoms of overdose.

TOLNAFTATE WITH TRICLOSAN

This combination is used in the prevention and treatment of athlete's foot and other common fungal infections, such as pityriasis versicolor. It is not recommended for use in deep nail bed or hair follicle infections.

How Tolnaftate with Triclosan Works

Tolnaftate acts to inhibit the growth of certain spores, but is not active against candida infections. Triclosan is a bis-phenol disinfectant, which is active against gram-positive and most gram-negative bacteria. It is used in surgical scrubs, soaps, and deodorants; it also controls staphylococcus germs.

Recommended Dosage

Apply to the infected area according to package instructions.

Side Effects of Tolnaftate with Triclosan

There have been isolated reports of skin irritation, redness, and pruritis when using tolnaftate with triclosan.

TRANSVASIN CREAM*

Transvasin cream is a skin ointment used for relief of itching, sunburn, muscular aches and pains, lumbago, rheumatism and fibrositis, as well as for treatment of minor cuts, scrapes, and burns. The ingredients (ethyl nicotinate, hexl nicotinate, tetrahydrofurfuryl salicylate, and benzocaine) work in combination to reduce pain and help minimize inflammation.

How Transvasin Works

All of the ingredients are local pain relievers, commonly used in a topical ointment. They are absorbed through the skin and reach the nerve fibers to temporarily block the conduction of the sensation of pain or discomfort to the brain. Benzocaine is a common surface anesthetic with a generally low toxicity.

Recommended Dosage

Use the smallest amount necessary to be effective. Follow label instructions and use as needed, applying cream to affected area and massaging gently until cream is absorbed. Apply no more than once per hour. Use caution when applying to children, as the ingredients are more likely to be absorbed into the system.

Side Effects of Transvasin

This cream is intended for external use only. People who are allergic to benzocaine or any of the other ingredients should not use this product. Do not use if you have a skin infection at the site of the treatment or if you have had severe or extensive skin disorders such as eczema or psoriasis.

TRIMETHOPRIM-SULFAMETHOXAZOLE
(Bioprim, Bactrim, Septra)

These two antibiotics have a wide spectrum of antibacterial activity. They are effective against uncomplicated urinary tract infections; sexually transmitted diseases such as gonorrhea; bronchitis, skin infections, toxoplasmosis, respiratory infections, and some AIDS-related infections such as *Pneumoncystis carinii* pneumonia, as well as genitourinary tract infections and gastrointestinal infections.

How Trimethoprim-Sulfamethoxazole Works

The two antibiotics that make up this drug work together by interfering with the life processes of bacteria at two crucial stages of development. The combination of sulfa and trimethoprim was an important advance in the development of antibiotics. The double-acting effect minimizes bacterial resistance. This makes the combination more effective than either drug alone, since bacteria immune to the action of one antibiotic can still be killed by the action of the other.

Recommended Dosage

The usual adult dosage is 960 milligrams twice daily by mouth for five days. Lower doses are indicated for long-term therapy and in patients with kidney impairment. The dosage for children is generally: age six weeks to five months, 120 milligrams twice daily; age six months to five years, 240 milligrams; six to twelve years, 480 milligrams. For serious infections, dosages may be higher and methods of administration should be determined by a physician.

Side Effects of Trimethoprim-Sulfamethoxazole

Adverse reactions may include nausea, vomiting, diarrhea, rashes, sensitivity to light, and dermatitis ranging from mild to severe. People with AIDS often react to this drug with fever, malaise, and rash.

VERAPAMIL HYDROCHLORIDE

Verapamil hydrochloride is a calcium-channel blocker, used to treat disturbances in heart rhythm and angina pectoris. It is also used to treat high blood pressure, asthma, and Raynaud's disease. It has been considered for use in manic-depressive disorder and migraine headache.

How Verapamil Hydrochloride Works

Verapamil hydrochloride is a member of a relatively new class of drugs that block the passage of calcium into the heart and smooth muscle, reducing heart contractions and need for oxygen by that muscle. Verapamil hydrochloride also widens or dilates the vessels bringing blood into the heart, thereby giving the heart a richer supply of oxygen-bearing blood. Thus, it increases the capacity to do physical exercise and reduces the pain of angina as well.

Recommended Dosage

Dosages vary depending upon the condition being treated. The usual dose is 240 to 480 milligrams per day in divided doses, taken one hour before or two hours after meals.

Side Effects of Verapamil Hydrochloride

The most common side effect is constipation. Some cases of abnormal liver function have also been reported. Other people experienced lowering of blood pressure, slowed heartbeat, dizziness, confusion, tingling in the arms and legs, headache, nausea, light-headedness, weakness, and fatigue from this drug. Additional side effects may include shakiness, muscle cramps, spotty menstruation, hair loss, and leg pains.

Using Verapamil Hydrochloride in Combination with Other Drugs

People taking verapamil hydrochloride will probably need to have their intake of digitalis lowered. Disopyramide should not be taken within forty-eight hours of taking verapamil, and taking calcium may interfere with the effectiveness of verapamil.

VIDARABINE PHOSPHATE

Vidarabine phosphate is an antiviral drug used in the treatment of herpes simplex keratitis. It has also been used in the treatment of chicken pox, Creutzfeld-Jacob disease, cytomegalovirus and cytomegalovirus retinitis, kidney failure, Epstein-Barr infections, infectious mononucleosis, encephalitis, hepatitis, and neonatal herpes simplex.

How Vidarabine Phosphate Works

Vidarabine phosphate appears to work by interfering in the early stages of the viral DNA synthesis, but the action may be more complex even than that. There is some evidence that it may inhibit other enzymes necessary to the virus's functioning and actually incorporate itself into the virus, destroying it from within. This drug does cross the blood-brain barrier, and is therefore useful in treating brain infections such as encephalitis.

Recommended Dosages

Vidarabine is applied as a 3 percent eye cream to treat herpes simplex retinitis and can be used when there has been no response to treatment with other antiviral drugs such as idoxuridine, or when there has been hypersensitivity or eye irritation with other drugs. The ointment is applied five times daily every three hours until the skin has healed, then twice daily for another seven days to prevent recurrence. It there is no healing within seven days or if complete healing has not occurred within twenty-one days, another form of therapy should be considered.

Side Effects of Vidarabine Phosphate

Adverse effects may occur when vidarabine is applied to the eyes. These include superficial punctate keratitis, sensitivity to light, tearing, and obstruction of the tear ducts.

Using Vidarabine in Combination with Other Drugs

Combinations of vidarabine and other antivirals such as Acyclovir have been found to work together well without increasing drug toxicity in vitro against cytomegalovirus and herpes simplex virus.

VINCAMINE

Vincamine is used to treat a variety of cerebral disorders such as psychiatric disturbances in the elderly, acute stroke, and cerebrovascular insufficiency.

How Vincamine Works

Vincamine and its salts are said to increase cerebral circulation and utilization of oxygen, thus making the brain work more efficiently.

Recommended Dosage

Vincamine is given by mouth in 40 to 80 milligram dosages.

Side Effects of Vincamine

Vincamine may have adverse effects on the cardiovascular system, and it should be taken with care by people who have high blood pressure or who have heart conditions.

WARFARIN

Warfarin is used to thin the blood and reduce the incidence of thrombosis or blood clots. It has no effect on existing blood clots but helps prevent new ones from forming. It is used to prevent and manage deep-vein blood clotting, formation of blood clots in the heart and lungs, preventing stroke and heart attack. Warfarin may be of some benefit in the treatment of lung cancer.

How Warfarin Works

Warfarin is an anticoagulant, which works by depressing the body's normal production of ingredients of the clotting process. Therefore, the blood becomes thinner, and the chance of blood clots in the arms, legs, lungs, heart, or brain is reduced.

Recommended Dosage

The dosage of warfarin you take must be closely regulated by your doctor. Your doctor will want to measure the time it takes for your blood to coagulate in order to regulate your dosage.

Side Effects of Warfarin

The major danger with warfarin is hemorrhage (uncontrolled bleeding), since your blood does not clot normally when you are taking it. Anemia or the formation of hematomas may occur. Side effects not necessarily associated with bleeding include baldness, fever, nausea, vomiting, diarrhea, priapism, and skin reactions.

Using Warfarin in Combination with Other Drugs

Many drugs interact with warfarin, including antibiotics, mineral oil, alcohol, aspirin, vitamin C, vitamin K, cholestyramine, phenylbutazone, oxyphenylbutazone, clofibrate, indomethacin, sulfa drugs, chloral hydrate, ethacrynic acid, mefenamic acid, nalidixic acid, tolbutamide, chlorpropamide, tolazamide, chloramphenicol, allopurinol, nortriptyline, methylphenidate, cimetidine, disulfiram, chlortetracycline, quinidine, haloperidol, MAO inhibitors, meperidine, thyroid hormones, antithyroid drugs, estrogens, steroids, griseofulvin, ethchlorvynol, meprobamate, costicosteroids, phenytoin, carbamazepine, and rifampin, propylthiouracil, and methylthiouracil.

Since this is only a partial list of potential drug interactions, patients should be carefully monitored. Also many green, leafy vegetables contain large amounts of vitamin K, a clotting agent which will reduce the effects of warfarin.

CHAPTER VIII

New Drugs under Investigation by the FDA and Not Yet Approved for Sale in the United States

The following is a list of some of the generic medications that are under investigation by the FDA. Depending on the results of testing, these drugs may become available in the United States. However, some of these medications have already received approval in other countries and are available by mail order importation.

By the time you read this book some of these drugs may have been approved by the FDA, but don't count on it. As I said before, unless there is strong political activity calling for action as in the case of AIDS drugs, don't expect this process to move very fast. Count on most of the drugs on this list to still be on it next year and the year after.

People who have conditions that could be affected by these medications may wish to check with their physician about the potential value of importing drugs that are still under investigation in this country. Please note that most of these drugs are not listed in the sample price lists at the end of Appendix I. Interested readers should contact some of the listed suppliers at the beginning of Appendix I to check availability.

ACECAINIDE (N-acetylprocainamide, NAPA, and acetylprocainamide)

Acecainide is helpful in treating irregular heartbeat or cardiac arrhythmias, especially premature ventricular complexes (PVCs) and refractory ventricular arrhythmias. There have been laboratory studies that suggest acecainide may be useful in converting atrial flutter to sinus rhythm.

In clinical trials, 63 percent of patients whose ventricular arrhythmias had not responded to other medication were under control within twelve months.

How Acecainide Works

Acecainide is a compound of procainamide, another cardiac medication, but it has properties that differ a great deal from its parent compound. Acecainide is classified as a type III antiarrhythmic agent, along with amariodone and bretylium, because of its ability to prolong atrial and ventricular action without substantial depression of conduction velocity. Other functions of the heart are not disturbed by the action of this drug.

Recommended Dosages

The usual dosage of acecainide is 500 milligrams every six to eight hours, but it may be adjusted up to 2.5 grams every eight hours.

Side Effects of Acecainide

The most common side effect of acecainide is nausea and vomiting; other side effects noted have included dizziness, light-headedness, blurred vision, numbness, and tingling. The lupuslike syndrome which frequently restricts the use of procainamide has not been observed with acecainide, making this drug preferable for many people. Like all antiarrhythmics, this drug may actually have an arrhythmia-inducing effect on some people.

ASTEMIZOLE

This drug is used in treating hay fever, allergic rhinitis, and any other conditions and allergies that benefit from antihistamine therapy.

How Astemizole Works

Astemizole is a long-acting, nonsedating histamine antagonist that is chemically unrelated to other antihistamines. Its major metabolite is desmethylastemizole.

Recommended Dosage

A daily dose of 10 milligrams is recommended. In people with severe symptoms, a regimen of 30 milligrams daily for up to seven days, followed by 10 milligrams daily has been suggested. Astemizole should be taken on an empty stomach.

Side Effects of Astemizole

Astemizole has a long period of effectiveness. Its need for only one dose per day plus a low incidence of side effects make this a promising drug for treating allergies. However, there is a rather long interval between taking the drug and symptom relief. This drug is most beneficial to people who are in need of long-term therapy.

BUPROPION

This drug has an antidepressant action that is useful in treating severe depression, simple depressed mood, cognitive impairments, insomnia, somatization, anxiety, and psychomotor retardation. Improvements have been particularly noted in cases of cognitive disturbances and where there was the presence of somatic complaints.

How Bupropion Works

Bupropion is a second generation antidepressant, chemically different from the common tricyclic antidepressants and more closely related to amphetamine. Its mechanism of action is not yet fully understood. However, it is known that this drug works in a way that does not affect the standard antidepressant pathways. Therefore, it can be used in conjunction with other antidepressants.

Recommended Dosage

Recommended levels vary depending on the nature of the illness. A starting dosage of 300 milligrams taken twice daily is commonly recommended.

Side Effects of Bupropion

The main adverse side effect is a relatively high rate of seizures among users. Other side effects include drowsiness during the day, cardiotoxicity, anticholinergic and antihistamine effects. However, some people have reported adverse reactions such as weight loss, dry mouth, and dizziness. Rare side effects include increased motor activity, tremor, excitement, agitation, insomnia, blurred vision, constipation, nausea, vomiting, urticaria, pruritus, rapid heartbeat, EEG abnormalities, headache, and sweating.

Using Bupropion in Combination with Other Drugs

When bupropion has been given experimentally along with tranquilizers in the benzodiazepine family or with alcohol, it abolished drowsiness and sedation, but does not alter feelings of alcohol inebriation.

CIFENLINE SUCCINATE

Cifenline succinate is used to treat heart arrhythmias, including a variety of ventricular arrhythmias, such as complex PVCs and nonsustained ventricular tachycardia.

How Cifenline Works

Cifenline is a new antiarrhythmic agent, which is derived from the drug imidazoline. Its effects are similar to those produced by quinidine, but response rates are higher than with quinidine. Over the long term, from 36 to 80 percent of people taking this drug have been helped.

Recommended Dosage

Cifenline appears to be a long-acting drug, so the frequency of dosage can be reduced. The starting dose is usually 130 milligrams, gradually increasing to 260 to 390 milligrams daily. People with impaired kidney function or kidney failure should take this drug in reduced dosages, as should older people.

Side Effects of Cifenline Succinate

Cifenline appears to be generally well tolerated by most people, especially in comparison to other antiarrhythmia drugs. Side effects reported include gastrointestinal complaints, light-headedness, dizziness, nervousness, tremulousness, blurred vision, and dry mouth. In some people it has worsened left ventricular dysfunction and should be used with caution by people who have a baseline ejection fraction of less than 30 percent.

DOMPERIDONE

Domperidone is used to treat nausea and vomiting, especially that which is induced by chemotherapy. It has also been used to treat ulcers, gastroesophageal reflux, and postoperative or bromocriptine-induced nausea and vomiting. Domperidone has been compared favorably to cimetidine in treating people with gastric ulcers as well as those with other gastrointestinal conditions.

Domperidone is effective against the severe and serious toxic nauseas that are common among cancer patients undergoing chemotherapy. This nausea and vomiting can be so severe that it interferes with therapy and nutrition. Domperidone seems to have fewer adverse side effects than current antinausea medications.

In studies of patients with Hodgkin's disease, domperidone decreased the duration of nausea and vomiting by greater than one-third when it was injected one hour before the start of chemotherapy. Higher dosages of domperidone did not achieve proportionally greater therapeutic response.

How Domperidone Works

This drug works by blocking the dopamine receptors. However, its primary benefit is that it does not cross the blood-brain barrier, thus has fewer central nervous system side effects such as drowsiness. It also interferes less with the normal workings of the intestine than other antinausea medications.

Recommended Dosage

The optimum dosage for the treatment of ulcers is 10 milligrams three times daily, about thirty minutes after a meal.

Side Effects of Domperidone

Domperidone has not been shown to produce significant side effects or toxicities. At higher dosages, patients have reported facial flushing, headache, slight sleepiness, and dry mouth. There have been isolated reports of some idiosyncratic extrapyramidal effects. Domperidone does not stimulate aldosterone secretion.

ENOXACIN

Enoxacin is an antibacterial drug used to treat infections such as *Pseudomonas aeruginosa* and uncomplicated urinary tract infections. It has frequently produced a better response than antibacterial drugs such as trimethoprim and sulfamethoxazole, augmentin and nitrofurantoin. Enoxacin has also been used to treat sexually transmitted diseases such as uncomplicated gonorrhea.

How Enoxacin Works

Enoxacin is a fluoroquinolone-related antimicrobial agent that is related to nalidixic acid, as well as norfloxacin and ciprofloxacin. It works by inhibiting the action of the bacterial DNA enzymes, as well as inhibiting RNA synthesis at higher dosages.

Recommended Dosage

The usual adult dosage is 400 to 600 milligrams twice daily. However, the dosage should be adjusted in people with kidney failure and in the elderly.

Side Effects of Enoxacin

The side effects of enoxacin seem to depend on the size of the dose and the duration of therapy. Those most frequently reported include nausea, vomiting, and diarrhea. Also noted in the laboratory were occurrences of elevated liver enzyme levels, eosinophilia, leukopenia, and neutropenia. Enoxacin has been shown to significantly inhibit the elimination of caffeine in some patients.

ERYTHROPOIETIN RECOMBINANT

Erythropoietin is a product of recombinant DNA technology and was granted orphan status in 1986. This new drug is being used for the anemia that usually accompanies end-stage kidney disease and in kidney dialysis patients. The use of erythropoietin makes transfusions, with their attendant risks, unnecessary. This drug is also used to eliminate the need for anabolic steroids in the treatment of kidney dialysis patients.

How Erythropoietin Works

Naturally occurring erythropoietin stimulates the rate of red blood cell production. It is normally produced in the kidneys and the liver, and it acts on certain cells in the bone marrow, causing the production of red cells. The recombinant replaces the erythropoietin that is not produced due to the kidney disease.

Recommended Dosage

Erythropoietin is administered intravenously in doses of 5 to 500 units per kilogram of body weight, three times weekly.

Side Effects of Erythropoietin

Erythropoietin has been well tolerated in clinical trials. Most side effects have been a result of the underlying disease rather than the treatment. Following injection, some people experienced pain or discomfort in their limbs and pelvis. Coldness and sweating without accompanying fever, within two hours of injection and persisting for up to twelve hours, was reported in four out of ten patients in one study. The increase in hematocrit was accompanied with a feeling of well-being in patients with end-stage kidney disease. Other side effects include raised blood pressure, iron deficiency, and elevated platelet counts.

ETODOLAC

Etodolac is a nonsteroidal analgesic as well as an anti-inflammatory, which shows value in relieving postoperative pain and the pain associated with arthritis, gout, menstruation, and ankylosing spondylitis.

How Etodolac Works

Etodolac works by preventing the sensitization of pain receptors and chemically inhibits the process of inflammation. In clinical studies it has proven valuable in relieving many types of pain, and in some respects is superior to aspirin because of its fewer side effects.

Recommended Dosage

The clinical dosages have ranged from 50 milligrams, the lowest effective dose, to 76 to 100 milligrams, which is comparable to 650 milligrams of aspirin and has a comparable duration of action from four to six hours. Single doses of 200 to 400 milligrams may produce a longer duration of effect, approximately six to eight hours.

Side Effects of Etodolac

Etodolac appears to be well tolerated in general. No significant side effects on kidney and liver function have been reported at present. Etodolac's primary benefit is that the gastrointestinal complaints and bleeding that are common with aspirin have not been reported with this drug.

FENOTEROL HBr

Fenoterol is used in preventing exercise-induced bronchospasm and acute attacks of mild to moderate asthma, and as maintenance therapy for chronic asthma or chronic obstructive lung disease.

How Fenoterol Works

Fenoterol dilates the bronchial tubes.

Recommended Dosage

The usual adult dosage is 200 to 400 micrograms, inhaled. Fenoterol has been available outside the United States for years in an inhaler, as an oral solution, and in powdered form.

Side Effects of Fenoterol

Side effects are rare, but include muscle tremor, tachycardia, palpitations, and nervousness.

FLURBIPROFEN

Flurbiprofen has been shown to be a safe and effective analgesic and anti-inflammatory in the treatment of rheumatoid arthritis, osteoarthritis, ankylosing spondylitis, acute gouty arthritis, shoulder tendonitis-bursitis, postpartum uterine pain, dental pain, painful menstruation, cancer pain, and pain secondary to soft tissue trauma. It has been used topically to treat excessive ultraviolet radiation exposure.

How Flurbiprofen Works

The efficacy of flurbiprofen has been compared to aspirin, acetaminophen with codeine, and other analgesics. It is of the same family as ibuprofen and naproxen. It has anti-inflammatory action and decreases the flow of blood into inflamed tissue.

Recommended Dosage

The analgesic dose for mild to moderate pain is 50 milligrams every four to six hours. For the treatment of inflammatory diseases such as arthritis, the usual dosage is 100 to 200 milligrams per day in two to four divided doses. Acute gouty arthritis has been treated with an initial 400 milligram loading dose in the first twenty-four hours, followed by 200 milligrams per day.

Side Effects of Flurbiprofen

Flurbiprofen is well tolerated at doses of 150 and 200 milligrams per day. The most frequent side effects have been mild abdominal discomfort and indigestion. The gastric changes are similar to those of ibuprofen. People with asthma, a history of upper gastrointestinal disturbances, and gastroesophageal reflux should use this drug with caution.

Using Flurbiprofen in Combination with Other Drugs

This drug may decrease the therapeutic effect of certain antihypertensive drugs. It may also displace oral hypoglycemics and benzodiazepines from their binding sites, delay the absorption of digoxin and antagonize the diuretic action of frusemide.

ISOXICAM

Isoxicam is a member of the oxicam class of drugs. It is used in the treatment of common rheumatic disorders such as rheumatoid arthritis and degenerative joint disease.

How Isoxicam Works

Isoxicam has potent and prolonged antipyretic, analgesic, and anti-inflammatory activity. Like the salicylates such as aspirin, it has an anticoagulant effect. In controlled studies, it has been found to be superior to aspirin in controlling the pain and inflammation of degenerative joint diseases and enhancing the freedom of movement. Isoxicam has been shown to reduce morning stiffness and relieve pain with relatively fewer side effects than other common remedies.

Recommended Dosage

A once daily dose of 200 milligrams is recommended.

Side Effects of Isoxicam

Isoxicam has been generally well tolerated and has caused few problems other than gastrointestinal effects. Other less commonly reported side effects include headache, dizziness, and ringing in the ears. There have been some incidences of skin reactions as well.

Using Isoxicam in Combination
with Other Drugs

Since this is an anticoagulant, it is not recommended to use aspirin along with this drug. The combination may increase gastrointestinal bleeding. Also isoxicam increases the anticoagulant action of warfarin.

KETOROLAC

Ketorolac is a nonsteroidal anti-inflammatory drug with pain-relieving and antipyretic activity. It is an analgesic used to control pain after childbirth, orthopedic postoperative pain, and other types of postsurgical pain.

How Ketorolac Works

Most scientists agree that this class of drugs works by inhibiting the synthesis of prostaglandins, natural body chemicals which affect the body's ability to feel pain.

Recommended Dosage

A single dose of 10 milligrams or 10 milligrams four times daily is considered comparable to, or even more effective than, 650 milligrams of aspirin. Its peak analgesic effect occurs three hours after administration.

Side Effects of Ketorolac

Few side effects have been reported. However, there have been rare reports of gastrointestinal irritation, fever, headache, and sleepiness.

KETOTIFEN

This drug is used in the treatment of asthma and the prevention of bronchospasms that are associated with asthma. Asthma is a chronic respiratory disease characterized by episodes of airway obstruction caused by a spasm of the bronchial tubes. The factors responsible for asthma are poorly understood. Some attacks are brought on by allergic reactions. Bronchodilators, such as ketotifen, counteract the bronchoconstrictive effects of the allergens.

How Ketotifen Works

Ketotifen has significant antihistamine and antiallergic properties that are useful in preventing asthma attacks before they occur. The introduction of the drug cromolyn marked the beginning of true prophylactic or preventive therapy for asthma attacks. Ketotifen appears to act in the same way as cromolyn. However, unlike cromolyn, which must be inhaled, ketotifen can be administered orally. It is well absorbed orally and its effects are sustained for up to twelve hours.

Recommended Dosage

One milligram orally, twice daily has been found to be effective in preventing and treating allergic asthma. Several weeks of administration are required in order to note improvement, and the patient must tolerate marked drowsiness. However, ketotifen does offer the convenience of oral administration.

Side Effects of Ketotifen

The most frequently reported side effects are sedation and drowsiness, which may require dosage reduction or discontinuation if the severity does not abate after continued therapy. Alcohol may increase these adverse reactions. Weight gain, dry mouth, headache, dizziness, and giddiness have also been reported.

Overdoses of ketotifen resulted in mild stomach pain, confusion, hyperexcitability, slowed heartbeat, rapid heartbeat, shortness of breath, convulsions, and unconsciousness, among others.

L-5 HYDROXYTRYPTOPHAN (L-5HTP)

L-5HTP is used for the treatment of postanoxic intention myoclonus. Myoclonus is a neuromuscular movement disorder characterized by involuntary, irregular muscle contractions. It is caused by brain lesions. L-5HTP has also shown some promise in treating depression and in preventing migraine.

How L-5HTP Works

Some of these irregular muscle contractions are related to brain neurotransmitter levels, especially those involving serotonin. L-5HTP is an aromatic amino acid which is the immediate precursor of serotonin. L-5HTP is administered along with carbidopa, a body chemical which decreases the conversion of L-5HTP to serotonin in the tissues. This permits a lower dose of L-5HTP to be given. Most people experienced an improvement of 50 percent or more from this treatment, including people with head trauma, methyl bromide toxicity, progressive myoclonus epilepsy, essential myoclonus, and palatal myoclonus.

Recommended Dosage

Beginning dose is 25 milligrams four times daily, increased by 100 milligrams per day every day, for three to five days, if there are no significant gastrointestinal side effects. A reduction in myoclonus is usually observed first at 600 to 1000 milligrams. The usual optimal dose of L-5HTP is between 1000 and 2000 milligrams per day in four divided doses.

Side Effects of L-5HTP

The most common side effects are loss of appetite, nausea, diarrhea, and vomiting. These can usually be avoided or minimized by gradual increases in the dosage of L-5HTP. The side effects rapidly disappear when the dosage is reduced or discontinued.

Rarer side effects include mental changes, such as euphoria that may progress to hypomania, restlessness, rapid speech, anxiety, insomnia, aggressiveness and agitation, mydriasis, light-headedness, sleepiness, blurring of vision, and slowed heartbeat. People with psychiatric disorders should not take L-5HTP because of its emotional side effects, although mental depression has been improved while on L-5HTP. Dyspnea sometimes accompanied by hyperventilation and light-headedness has also been reported. L-5HTP should not be used by people who have kidney disease, peptic ulcer, platelet disorders, scleroderma, and Parkinson's disease. This drug may unmask a scleroderma condition.

Using L-5HTP in Combination with Other Drugs

MAO (monoamine oxidase) inhibitors and reserpine should not be taken concurrently with this drug. Fenfluramine releases brain serotonin and may potentiate this treatment.

MILRINONE

Milrinone is used in the treatment of patients with severe congestive heart failure. It has positive inotropic and vasodilator qualities and appears to be very well tolerated. Milrinone has shown nearly twenty times the therapeutic potency of amrinone, the parent compound. Milrinone has the ability to increase the contractile force of the heartbeat and increase the heart output with only a minimum increase in heart rate.

Other favorable effects include significant reductions in left-ventricular and diastolic blood pressure, pulmonary wedge pressure, right atrial pressure, systemic vascular resistance, and a slight reduction of mean arterial pressure.

How Milrinone Works

Milrinone increases the oxygen utilization of the heart, expands the blood vessels, and enhances the efficiency of the failing heart.

Recommended Dosage

A typical dose is likely to be 5 or 10 milligrams every three or four hours. Experts feel that a time-release version of this drug needs to be developed before it goes into widespread use.

Side Effects of Milrinone

In contrast to digitalis glycosides, milrinone is relatively nontoxic. In fact, it appears to be relatively free of adverse side effects. With chronic oral use, there have been reports of headaches and some worsening of angina pectoris. However, all of these cases had underlying coronary artery disease.

MISOPROSTOL

Misoprostol is an antiulcer drug for people who have failed to respond to drugs such as cimetidine and Zantac.

Conditions such as esophagitis, acute hemorrhagic gastritis, and aspirin- or alcohol-induced gastritis may also be treatable by this drug.

How Misoprostol Works

Misoprostol inhibits the secretion of gastric acids. In addition to an antisecretory effect, misoprostol also has a cyto-protective or mucosal-protective effect. How it does this is still not understood, but misoprostol seems to increase the production of gastric mucosa, thicken the mucosal gel layer, and increase the blood flow to the mucosa to aid in the repair of damaged tissues.

Recommended Dosage

Doses of 200 micrograms taken four times daily have been shown to be as effective as 300 milligrams of cimetidine taken four times daily.

Side Effects of Misoprostol

Diarrhea is the most common side effect; nausea and vomiting were also infrequently reported.

NITRENDIPINE

Nitrendipine is a vasodilator used to treat mild to moderate high blood pressure, especially low renin hypertension, which accounts for 20 to 30 percent of the hypertensive population.

Preliminary studies suggest that this drug has no effect on blood glucose, total cholesterol, triglyceride, or uric acid levels. It does not alter the kidney function and has a short-term diuretic effect.

How Nitrendipine Works

Nitrendipine is a potent vasodilator that may represent an improvement over other currently used antihypertensive drugs because of its lower incidence of undesirable side effects. It causes a decrease in both systolic and diastolic blood pressure. Nitrendipine is classified as a type II calcium antagonist, structurally similar to nifedipine. Relaxation of blood vessels occurs as a result of inhibiting calcium influx against cellular membranes.

Recommended Dosage

The initial recommended dose is 5 to 20 milligrams daily, taken in the morning, after ingestion of food, then increased between 5 to 20 milligrams, twice daily as needed.

Side Effects of Nitrendipine

The side effect most frequently reported is headache. Fatigue, peripheral edema, flushing, palpitations, and mild elevations in liver function have also been reported. Nitrendipine may precipitate myocardial ischemia in people with coronary artery disease. There have been reflex increases in heart rate, AV nodal conduction, and myocardial contractility.

OMEPRAZOLE

Omeprazole is an inhibitor of gastric acid secretion and promises to be especially helpful in treating people with Zollinger-Ellison syndrome and others who do not respond to drugs such as cimetidine.

People with gastric ulcers have been shown to obtain comparable healing rates whether on omeprazole, Zantac, or cimetidine. People with reflux esophagitis who took omeprazole once daily responded with higher rates of complete healing than those who took Zantac twice daily. For people with Zollinger-Ellison syndrome that was unresponsive to cimetidine or Zantac therapy, high doses of omeprazole caused complete inhibition of gastric acid secretion and brought about symptomatic improvements for the duration of therapy.

How Omeprazole Works

Gastric acid is secreted as a response to three different stimuli: cholinergic, histaminergic, and gastrinergic. Chemically, omeprazole seems to act by blocking gastric acid secretion to a 90 percent greater extent than H_2 blockers. Direct application of omeprazole to the gastric mucosa seems to produce a cyto-protective effect, defending the tissue against erosion by acids. The duration of this protective effect is much shorter, however, than the effect of inhibiting the acid production itself.

Recommended Dosage

Omeprazole is usually given in doses of 20 to 40 milligrams once daily.

Side Effects of Omeprazole

In short-term trials of four to eight weeks for acute ulcer disease, omeprazole appears to be well tolerated. Side effects reported include diarrhea, nausea, dry mouth, dizziness, weakness, headache, and numbness.

PINACIDIL

This is a new drug used for the treatment of high blood pressure or hypertension. The action of pinacidil is comparable to other cardiac medications such as minoxidil, guancydine, and diazoxide. However, compared to another hydralazine, pinacidil is more potent and effective in lowering blood pressure. It also produces less of an increase in myocardial oxygen consumption than with hydralazine. Pinacidil has been particularly effective in patients with kidney impairment.

How Pinacidil Works

Pinacidil acts at the level of the precapillary vessels, causing reduction in the resistance of vascular smooth muscle. It has a vasodilator effect.

Recommended Dosage

The most effective dose range appears to be 12.5 to 25 milligrams twice daily. Some physicians feel that the drug requires three times daily administration.

Side Effects of Pinacidil

Pinacidil appears to be well tolerated. There have only been a few reports of dizziness, headache, and facial flushing. The incidence of edema ranges from about 24 to 46 percent, so diuretics may have to be taken concurrently by most people.

Since this drug is excreted by the liver, people with impaired liver function need to have their therapy initiated slowly, at low doses and with constant monitoring. Pinacidil seems to be safe and effective, with moderate to severe hypertension, especially when added to a regimen of a diuretic and beta blocker.

PIRENZEPINE HYDROCHLORIDE

This drug is used for the treatment of ulcers, including duodenal ulcers and peptic ulcers. Pirenzepine hydrochloride is a tricyclic benzodiazepine antiulcer agent comparable to cimetidine and ranitidine.

Combined use of pirenzepine hydrochloride with cimetidine or ranitidine shows greater effect than using either one alone. This may make pirenzepine hydrochloride more useful in treating Zollinger-Ellison syndrome and peptic ulcer conditions that have been resistant to single drug therapy.

How Pirenzepine Hydrochloride Works

Pirenzepine hydrochloride has selective activity for gastric acid secretion. It suppresses both basal and pepsin secretion, with lesser effects on other acids, such as saliva.

Recommended Dosage

An initial dose of 50 milligrams, two to three times daily inhibits acid secretion for at least up to four to five hours. Higher dosages inhibit the esophageal and colonic motility, and decrease lower esophageal sphincter pressure. Dosage must be reduced when the patient has impaired kidney function, since this drug is mostly excreted by the kidneys.

Side Effects of Pirenzepine Hydrochloride

Pirenzepine hydrochloride is generally well tolerated, with few adverse side effects. Dry mouth is the most often reported side effect, but nausea, vomiting, diarrhea, constipation, increased appetite, anorexia, tiredness, and transient visual difficulties have all occurred. Daily doses of less than 150 milligrams have seemed to reduce some of these problems.

SUMATRIPTAN

Sumatriptan is a new drug that holds great promise in the treatment of migraine headaches. While this drug is still very new, early results have been encouraging for its widespread use. Two out of every three migraine sufferers who have used sumatriptan report relief from symptoms.

How Sumatriptan Works

Sumatriptan belongs to a new class of drugs that are known as serotonin blockers. These drugs act on neurotransmission in the brain, specifically on the neurotransmitter serotonin. Sumatriptan works to treat migraine because it blocks a group of serotonin receptors (called 5-HT1-like) that control the constriction of blood vessels leading into the brain.

Recommended Dosage

Early indications are that 100 milligrams taken at the onset of the migraine is easily tolerated and works about as well as larger doses.

Side Effects of Sumatriptan

The most commonly reported side effects are mild feelings of tingling, warmth and heaviness, and pressure on the chest. People who have a history of angina or ischemic heart disease should not use this drug.

CHAPTER IX

Sample Listing of Orphan Drugs Available Outside the United States

For purposes of this book, "orphan drugs" is the name that we are using for that group of drugs that have been approved for use in another country, but are neither marketed in the US nor approved by the FDA. Usually, this is because the FDA approval process is too expensive and the potential American market too small to make it financially profitable for a company to market such a drug.

In the following list of generic orphan drugs, I give you a small subset of those that are available in other parts of the world through mail order importation. For more complete information on this subject, consult your physician as well as Anderson and Anderson's *Orphan Drugs*. This list is only intended to provide a sample of what is on the market.

All the drugs in this chapter can be ordered by special request from the sources listed at the end of this book. If you have a rare disease that could benefit from one of these (or another orphan drug) talk to your doctor, and then call one of these sources. Please note that most of these drugs are not listed in the sample price lists at the end of Appendix I.

ACETYLDIGITOXIN

Acetyldigitoxin is useful for symptoms associated with serious heart problems. It encourages the heart to beat

175

more powerfully and efficiently. The action of acetyldigitoxin helps reduce the size of an enlarged heart, improves kidney functions, and encourages the body to get rid of excess fluid in the tissues (edema) which is associated with heart failure. Each beat of the heart is made more efficient by acetyldigitoxin and therefore fewer heartbeats are needed to accomplish the heart's work. Rapid heartbeat (tachycardia) is also reduced by this drug.

How Acetyldigitoxin Works

The major component of acetyldigitoxin is a well-known medication called digitalis. Digitalis is manufactured from the foxglove plant, an established heart remedy for many years. Acetyldigitoxin is an improvement on digitalis itself, since it remains in the body longer and is metabolized more slowly, thus increasing the term of effectiveness.

Digitalis-based drugs work by stimulating the heart to beat more forcefully and thus pump a greater volume of blood at each beat. This allows the blood to carry more oxygen to the brain and other tissues. These drugs also allow the heart to rest more completely between contractions.

Recommended Dosage

The usual dose of acetyldigitoxin is 100 to 200 micrograms per day for maintenance therapy, after an initial dosage of 800 micrograms to 1 milligram per day. Several hours may pass after dosage before its beneficial effects are noticed.

Calcium should be avoided when taking acetyldigitoxin, because calcium influences the action of all digitalis-based drugs and can even cause dangerous heart arrhythmias or fibrillation (loss of rhythmic heartbeat) when taken with these drugs.

Side Effects of Acetyldigitoxin

Side effects include loss of appetite, nausea, vomiting, skin rashes, and allergies such as pruritus and urticaria. Infrequently, people have experienced convulsions, disorientation, aphasia, and abnormal color vision.

Those who have a very slow heartbeat, a condition called bradycardia, should not use this drug since it tends to slow heartbeat even more. People with any condition such as Stokes-Adams syndrome should also avoid acetyldigitoxin, since blood flow to the brain could be interrupted by slowed heart function. People who are experiencing mineral imbalance or impaired kidney or liver functioning should use care in taking acetyldigitoxin as well.

ADENOSINE TRIPHOSPHATE

Adenosine triphosphate is a vasodilator, a drug that stimulates blood flow by expanding the veins and arteries. It is useful in helping treat abnormal heart rhythms and conditions associated with cardiac insufficiency.

The unique properties of this drug have made it of interest in treating muscular dystrophy. It has also been used with some success in the alleviation of stiff joints and pain associated with arthritis. Another potential use for adenosine triphosphate is to protect the body against chromosome damage. It is used for this purpose by people who work with X rays.

How Adenosine Triphosphate Works

Adenosine triphosphate is a natural constituent of animal cells. It is converted by the body to adenosine diphosate, releasing energy during the process. This energy stimulates cellular activity such as muscle contractions.

This drug helps increase muscular strength and increased blood circulation in the arms and legs, and stimulates a more efficient heartbeat. For elderly people, this results in more power in the muscles and a greater range of motion despite weakening muscles.

Recommended Dosage

The recommended dosage is two 3 milligram tablets, three times daily, totalling 18 milligrams per day, for one week. Following that, a maintenance dose of four to eight tablets daily is given.

Side Effects of Adenosine Triphosphate

No side effects have been reported for adenosine triphosphate as of the date of this publication.

ALPRENOLOL HYDROCHLORIDE

Alprenolol hydrochloride belongs to the family of drugs called beta blockers. It is used to treat high blood pressure, anxiety, irregular heart rhythms; it also helps to reduce the chance of a second heart attack. Increased physical demands on the heart are associated with the chest pain of angina pectoris, so this drug is helpful in alleviating angina as well.

How Alprenolol Works

Alprenolol actually causes the heart to require less oxygen to perform its work and thus reduces the effort the heart muscle must put forth. Beta blockers interfere with the nerve impulses that signal the heart to work harder during periods of stress. Thus the heart needs less oxygen and stresses itself less during activities such as physical exertion.

Recommended Dosage

Alprenolol comes in 50 and 100 milligram tablets. When treating angina and other conditions, 200 to 400 milligrams every day in divided doses is recommended. In alleviating high blood pressure, 200 milligrams per day is the initial dosage. This may be increased weekly up to 800 milligrams per day.

Side Effects of Alprenolol

Some of the reported side effects of alprenolol are nausea, headache, mild depression, sedation, dry mouth, dizziness, diarrhea, symptoms of angina, and a decreased sex drive.

People who have an abnormally slow heartbeat, hypoglycemia, metabolic acidosis, diabetes mellitus, bronchial asthma, heart block, or who are taking narcotics that affect or depress heart activity should not take this medication.

ANETHOLTRITHION

Anetholtrithion can be used to relieve dry mouth whether caused by medication or by radiation treatments. Some of the drugs which can cause dry mouth include anti-parkinsonism drugs and tranquilizers. Anetholtrithion also encourages the production of liver bile, which can help relieve nausea, flatus, distended abdomen, and poor digestion. Anetholtrithion has also been used to help dry eyes by encouraging the flow of tears.

How Anetholtrithion Works

This medication increases the flow of natural body liquids, such as tears, saliva, and liver bile, by directly stimulating the cells that produce these fluids.

Recommended Dosage

Anetholtrithion is available in 12.5 and 25 milligram tablets, and a 12.5 milligram dose in granule form. In treating the lack of saliva, the usual dosage is 75 milligrams per day in three divided doses, taken before each meal. In treating lack of sufficient bile, this medication is usually taken in divided doses, before meals, of 50 milligrams per day with ten to fifteen drug-free days each month.

Side Effects of Anetholtrithion

Diarrhea and softening of the feces have been noted, which is usually alleviated by reducing the dosage. People with liver or gall bladder abnormalities should not take this drug. This includes cirrhosis and liver canal, bile duct, or biliary tract obstruction. Pregnant women should not take this drug, since it has not proven to be safe for the developing fetus. Some research suggests that anetholtrithion may have an interaction with certain psychiatropic drugs.

ANTAZOLINE (PHENAZOLINE HYDROCHLORIDE)

Antazoline is used to alleviate sneezing, hay fever, runny nose, itching, insect bites, and other allergic reactions, as well as to suppress nausea. Antazoline is a short-term antihistamine, which is not as strong as other antihistamines, but makes up for it by having fewer side effects.

How Antazoline Works

Antazoline works by inhibiting smooth muscle responses to histamine and antagonizing the action of histamine that results in capillary permeability.

Recommended Dosage

Antazoline is available in 100 milligram tablets, as well as a nasal spray, eye drops, and a topical skin cream. Adult dose is one or two tablets every three to four hours after meals, not to exceed twelve tablets (1200 milligrams) in twenty-four hours. Do not take antazoline for more than five days at a time because there is a risk of rebound congestion. There is also a risk of overdose with the nasal spray, especially in children under five. This drug is sensitive to light and air and must be kept in a cool, dark place away from moisture.

Side Effects of Antazoline

Side effects reported include dry mouth, nausea, drowsiness, rashes, upset stomach, and urinary urgency. Children may become hyperactive when using this drug.

Antazoline may depress the central nervous system and can interact with many other drugs, such as alcohol, tranquilizers, and sedatives, causing depression of the nervous system. Hence caution is recommended when using this drug with any of the corticosteroids.

APROTININ

Aprotinin is mainly used for the treatment of hemorrhage (especially to lessen bleeding after stomach surgery), acute pancreatitis, arthritis, urticaria, and to support the therapeutic administration of insulin to diabetics.

How Aprotinin Works

Aprotinin works by blocking the action of various digestive enzymes, which may become overactive and interfere with the effects of insulin or else digest pancreatic tissue. Aprotinin is made from a substance found in the lungs of cows.

Recommended Dosage

Aprotinin is administered intravenously and dosage is expressed in kallikrein inactivator units. For the treatment of hemorrhage, up to 500,000 kallikrein units are administered by slow intravenous injection, followed by 200,000 units every hour by continuous infusion. Prior to upper abdominal surgery, 200,000 units are given by slow intravenous injection, followed by 200,000 units by continuous intravenous infusion, every four hours on the day of the operation and for the next two days.

Side Effects of Aprotinin

Some people react allergically with bronchospasm or skin rashes to this drug. Other side effects include nausea and diarrhea, difficulty in breathing, muscle pain, heart palpitations, and changes in blood pressure.

AZAPROPAZONE

This aspirinlike agent is used to relieve arthritic pain and inflammation, gout, ankylosing spondylitis, and other rheumatic disorders. This drug is related to anti-inflammatories such as phenylbutazone but has much milder side effects.

How Azapropazone Works

Azapropazone is an aspirinlike drug that works by inhibiting prostaglandin synthetase.

Recommended Dosage

Azapropazone is available in 300 milligram capsules and 800 milligram tablets. The average dose is 1200 milligrams daily in 300 milligram doses four times per day or 800 milligrams twice daily, after meals. For treating gout, 2400 milligrams daily in divided doses is recommended, and later lowered to 1200 milligrams in divided doses.

Side Effects of Azapropazone

Side effects include photosensitivity, stomach upset, kidney disorder, rashes, dizziness, and water retention. People with stomach disturbances such as peptic ulcers or who have impaired kidney functions should take this drug with great caution.

Using Azapropazone in Combination with Other Drugs

There may be a drug interaction with anticonvulsants, sulfa drugs, or diabetic medications. People with allergic reactions to aspirin and phenylbutazone should avoid azapropazone.

BENZARONE

Benzarone helps relieve disorders of the circulatory system such as varicose veins, fragile capillaries, phlebitis, and poor circulation in the legs. It is also used in the treatment of other conditions that involve impaired circulation such as high blood pressure, diabetes, hardening of the arteries (atherosclerosis), or hemorrhage.

How Benzarone Works

Benzarone strengthens the inner cell layer of the blood vessels, as well as helping dissolve blood clots.

Recommended Dosage

This drug may be applied as an ointment or taken as three 200 milligram tablets a day following a meal, for three weeks.

Side Effects of Benzarone

Benzarone has been known to cause upset stomach, diarrhea, skin rash, and allergic conjunctivitis.

BIETAMIVERINE HYDROCHLORIDE (DIETAMIVERINE DIHYDROCHLORIDE)

This drug treats pain that is caused by muscle spasms such as menstrual cramps, pain following childbirth, pain of both stomach and duodenal ulcer, spasms of the digestive tract and esophagus, kidney stones, and spastic colon.

How Bietamiverine Works

Bietamiverine acts on the smooth muscle tissue in the gastric and urinary tract, relaxing it and relieving the painful cramps of spasms.

Recommended Dosage

This drug is available in 50 milligram tablets and 100 milligram suppositories. It is taken as two or three tablets of 100 or 150 milligrams or one or two suppositories of 100 or 200 milligrams per day.

Side Effects of Bietamiverine

Not available at this time. Consult your physician or pharmacist for more information.

BORNAPRINE HYDROCHLORIDE

Bornaprine is an anti-parkinson drug that helps alleviate the tremors caused by the disease.

How Bornaprine Works

This drug is an antimuscarinic agent which has an antispasmodic effect on smooth muscles.

Recommended Dosage

The usual beginning dosage is one half tablet (2 milligrams) per day, which may be gradually increased to a maximum of 6 to 12 milligrams daily, if necessary, to relieve symptoms.

Side Effects of Bornaprine

Reported side effects include dry mouth, blurred vision, dizziness, rapid heartbeat, constipation, tiredness, dehydration, and difficulty in urinating. People who are suffering from acute glaucoma should avoid this drug, as should people with an intestinal obstruction or conditions such as megacolon.

BUFEXAMAC

This drug helps relieve skin conditions such as acne, eczema, topical and contact dermatitis, psoriasis, periphlebitis, pruritus, diaper rash, and folliculitis. It can also be used to alleviate inflammations of the genitals, rheumatoid arthritis, hemorrhoids, various other types of arthritis, mild burns, and insect bites.

How Bufexamac Works

When a tissue is injured, it releases chemicals that cause swelling, redness, and pain. Bufexamac (which is not a steroid) helps to reduce these manifestations, soothing inflammation and relieving the pain and oozing that often accompany skin disorders.

Recommended Dosage

Bufexamac is available in tubes as a cream or ointment. Rub bufexamac into the affected area two or three times a day.

Side Effects of Bufexamac

There may be burning or stinging when bufexamac is first applied. If allergic to this drug, a rash often occurs.

CIFENLINE SUCCINATE

Cifenline is a new cardiac drug used to alleviate ventricular and supraventricular arrhythmias. It may also be helpful in preventing these conditions.

How Cifenline Works

Cifenline works by interfering with the depolarization of the cardiac membrane through blocking the inward flow of sodium into the cardiac cells.

Recommended Dosage

The usual dosage of cifenline is 130 milligrams to start, then 4 to 6 milligrams per kilogram of body weight or 260 to 390 milligrams daily. People with reduced kidney functioning, such as the elderly, may require a lower dosage.

Side Effects of Cifenline

Known side effects include light-headedness and dry mouth, but this medication is usually well tolerated.

CHLORPHENTERMINE HYDROCHLORIDE

Chlorphentermine is used in weight-control programs, especially by diabetics to help control appetite. This drug is meant only to assist in short-term weight control. It is an anorectic (appetite depressant), used so that a person can more easily comply with dietary restrictions.

How Chlorphentermine Hydrochloride Works

Chlorphentermine hydrochloride works by stimulating the central nervous system, leading to a loss of interest in eating.

Recommended Dosage

Chlorphentermine is available as 65 milligram tablets. The usual dosage is one tablet either during or following the morning meal.

Side Effects of Chlorphentermine

This medication affects the ability of a person to drive and to operate machinery. It has also been shown to cause drowsiness, restlessness, headache, heart palpitations, dry mouth, rapid heartbeat, nausea, constipation, and difficulty in urination.

Chlorphentermine is not intended for children under fifteen, nor for nursing mothers or pregnant women. It is not recommended for those with high blood pressure, hyperthyroidism, angina pectoris, or glaucoma. There have been reports that it may adversely affect storage of fats in the blood and may be implicated in pulmonary hypertension.

CLOBETASONE BUTYRATE

This drug is used in alleviating sunburn, skin irritations, eczema, seborrheic dermatitis, and other skin irritations or eruptions. Clobetasone is of the corticosteroid family of drugs but is much stronger than over-the-counter hydrocortisone. However, it is less likely to create side effects such as skin atrophy in which the skin loses its elasticity and can become discolored.

Any steroid can be absorbed into the system from the site of application. This can cause the body to shut down production of its own natural corticosteroids, which can affect metabolism and many other body processes. It can take several months for the body to reestablish its normal function.

How Clobetasone Works

Clobetasone works like other steroids by inhibiting the body's inflammatory response.

Recommended Dosage

This drug is applied topically as an ointment or cream to the skin. It is also available in eyedrops. Spread the cream thinly over the irritated area two or three times per day and massage in gently. Do not exceed 100 grams per week.

After applying this drug, do not cover the area with a bandage or with plastic. This can cause systemic absorption. Do not apply this drug to herpes sores, tuberculous skin lesions, or to fungus infections such as candidiasis or moniliasis, vaccinia (cowpox). It should not be used in or near the eyes, unless in drop form.

Side Effects of Clobetasone

Side effects may include burning, itching, irritation, drying of the skin, secondary infections, and changes in skin color. People with impaired circulation, such as in conditions of stasis dermatitis, should not use this drug.

This drug should not be applied to a skin infection, unless an antibiotic is also being used for the infection. A characteristic of corticosteroids is that they may suppress the inflammation and manifestations of infection, but they do not attack the underlying cause of the infection itself.

CYCLOFENIL

This drug has been used in treating infertility caused by a failure to ovulate. It acts on the reproductive system; also it can relieve menstrual disorders such as scanty menstruation, menopausal discomforts, premenstrual syndrome, and cessation of menstruation. It can also help correct the menstrual cycle after long use of oral contraceptives. Cyclofenil is also useful in treating scleroderma (overly thick skin).

How Cyclofenil Works

This drug works on the female reproductive organs by inhibiting the effects of estrogen and then enlarging the size of the ovaries, and thus encouraging fertility.

Recommended Dosage

Cyclofenil is usually administered in doses of 100 milligrams, twice daily for three menstrual cycles, or for three months if menstruation is irregular.

Side Effects of Cyclofenil

Cyclofenil can cause hot flashes, enlargement of the ovaries, and gastric distress. Headaches, loss of appetite, and nausea have also been reported. Infrequently, occurrences of jaundice have occurred after using this drug. Women with severe or chronic liver disorders should avoid this medication.

DISOPROPYLAMINE DICHLORACETATE

This medication is useful in alleviating the symptoms of angina pectoris or Raynaud's phenomenon. It is also used in treatment of cerebrovascular disorders. Dichloracetate is taken to increase the flow of blood to the brain, arms, and legs.

How Disopropylamine Dichloracetate Works

This drug dilates blood vessels and thereby increases blood flow to the arms and legs, as well as brain. With the increased volume of blood comes more oxygen and other blood-borne nutrients.

Recommended Dosage

Usually this drug is taken as six 50 milligram tablets a day in divided doses of 100 milligrams each, followed by a maintenance dosage of three tablets a day for a month or three tablets per day every second or third day.

Side Effects of Disopropylamine Dichloracetate

Few side effects have been reported if the recommended dosage is followed.

ETOFYLLINE

Etofylline is useful in alleviating the symptoms of asthma and hyperlipidemia, a condition characterized by high fat levels in the blood. When treating cerebral ischemia, etofylline helps to relieve dizziness, visual problems, and behavioral irregularities that occur when the volume of blood to the brain is decreased.

How Etofylline Works

Etofylline works by dilating the blood vessels and thus allowing more blood to reach the brain. It is manufactured from a caffeinelike substance found in tea leaves. The drug is chemically similar to aminophylline, a heart stimulant which also lowers blood pressure, expands the bronchial tubes, and encourages greater oxygen circulation.

Recommended Dosage

Etofylline is available in 100 milligram tablets and suppositories. The recommended adult dosage is 300 to 500 milligrams per day by mouth or suppository. Pregnant women or children under fifteen should not take this medication.

Side Effects of Etofylline

Reported side effects include tachycardia (rapid heartbeat) and insomnia. A few cases of overdose have resulted in convulsions.

This drug should be used with caution by people with heart disease, peptic ulcers, liver impairment, hyperthyroidism, or epilepsy. Etofylline may interact with other medications, such as cimetidine and erythromycin.

FENCLOFENAC

Fenclofenac is used to relieve the pain and other symptoms of arthritis (including osteoarthritis, rheumatoid arthritis, and psoriatic arthritis), ankylosing spondylitis, synovitis, sciatica, and prolapsed vertebral discs.

Fenclofenac is far stronger than aspirin and has a similar action to ibuprofen. It is an anti-inflammatory drug that provides pain relief. Fenclofenac is nonsteroidal and is manufactured from phenylacetic acid.

How Fenclofenac Works

Fenclofenac works like other anti-inflammatories by inhibiting cyclooxygenose, which then reduces the synthesis of prostaglandins.

Recommended Dosage

The recommended adult dosage is two to four 300 milligram tablets daily, in divided doses, taken with food. The average maintenance dosage is three tablets per day.

It is not recommended for children, pregnant women, or nursing mothers.

Side Effects of Fenclofenac

This drug may cause upset stomach or other gastrointestinal complaints, blurred vision, skin rash, and headache. People who are allergic to aspirin, who have asthma, peptic ulcer, gastrointestinal lesions, liver or kidney dysfunction, or eczema should not take this medication.

FENTIAZAC

Fentiazac helps people with joint disorders. It is an anti-inflammatory drug that is used for rheumatoid arthritis, gouty arthritis, muscle and joint disorders, synovitis, tendonitis, bursitis, and spondylarthritis. It also reduces fever, pain, and inflammation and helps people to move their afflicted joints more easily and with less pain.

How Fentiazac Works

Fentiazac works on the chemical dysfunction that causes joint inflammation disorders and rheumatic diseases. It is not a steroid.

Recommended Dosage

This medication is supplied as tablet or a topical cream. The recommended dose depends on the condition of the patient and initial response to treatment. When taken orally, the typical dose is one or two 100 milligram tablets once or twice daily.

Side Effects of Fentiazac

Fentiazac is occasionally found to bring about symptoms of stomach upset and gastric distress.

FENTONIUM BROMIDE

This is a gastrointestinal medication that has proven useful in alleviating stomach conditions including eroding and recurrent ulcers, peptic ulcer, gastrointestinal spasms, benign stomach and duodenal ulcers, gastric erosion of the esophagus, and gastroduodenitis.

How Fentonium Bromide Works

This drug is classified as an anticholinergic. Like atropine, it works to reduce excess acidity and secretion of gastric fluids which are corrosive to the affected tissue. It also reduces excessive movement of the gastrointestinal tract. In treating ulcers, it seems to block certain chemical body functions that lead to the formation of ulcers.

Recommended Dosage

Fentonium is prescribed in 20 milligram tablets. For gastritis and related disorders, three tablets daily for three weeks is recommended. In relieving gastroduodenal ulcer, three to four tablets daily is recommended for the first week. This is usually followed by a reduction to three tablets daily for the next four weeks.

Side Effects of Fentonium Bromide

This family of anticholinergic drugs may be responsible for side effects that include difficulty in swallowing and urination, as well as dry mouth. They may also cause blurred vision that is a response to increased pressure in the eyeball. Dry skin, flushing, and heart palpitations may also be experienced. Constipation and tolerance to this drug may develop in certain people.

FLOCTAFENINE

Floctafenine is an anti-inflammatory drug that is used to relieve painful menstruation, joint pain such as that of arthritis and sciatica, bone and muscle pain associated with injury, pain that follows oral surgery, and even cancer pain.

How Floctafenine Works

This drug is believed to work against pain by lowering the volume of prostaglandins, body chemicals that contribute to the inflammatory response. Floctafenine is recommended only for short-term relief of pain.

Recommended Dosage

Floctafenine is available as 200 milligram tablets, which can be broken into smaller pieces. Most people take 200 to 400 milligrams three or four times per day as needed. Dosage should not exceed 1200 milligrams per day.

Side Effects of Floctafenine

The reported side effects of this drug include headache, nausea, diarrhea, drowsiness, dizziness, heartburn, constipation, gastrointestinal bleeding, difficulty in urinating, skin rashes, and insomnia. People with peptic ulcers and other severe inflammatory disorders should not take this drug. Caution should also be used by those with impaired kidney function, who have difficulty urinating, or who are taking anticoagulant medication.

FONAZINE MESYLATE

This antihistamine is used to treat allergic disorders, including dermatitis, hay fever, migraine headaches, rhinitis, urticaria, allergic eczema, seborrheic dermatitis pruritus, topical dermatitis, prurigo, and itching of the anogenital area. It is also useful in controlling bronchial asthma and motion sickness. Fonazine is less likely to cause drowsiness than other antihistamines.

How Fonazine Mesylate Works

It works by reducing the action of histamine, a body chemical that is responsible for many allergic reactions. Fonazine also acts against serotonin, which is thought to be implicated in the allergy process.

Recommended Dosage

Fonazine is available both in 20 milligram capsules and suppositories. Adults initially take one 20 milligram capsule three times daily, gradually increasing dosages to a total daily intake of 120 milligrams in three divided doses as needed.

Side Effects of Fonazine Mesylate

Reported side effects of this drug include drowsiness, confusion, dry mouth, blurred vision, dizziness, fatigue, skin rash, and nervousness. There may be some relief from these side effects at a lowered dosage. Do not use alcoholic beverages or operate machinery while using fonazine.

HEXAMETHYLMELAMINE

This is an anticancer drug used in the treatment of ovarian cancer and other solid tumors, as well as lung and cervical cancers.

How Hexamethylmelamine Works

Two other cancer-treating drugs in the same family are triethylenemalmine and tretamine. Hexamethylmelamine blocks the production of certain chemicals that the cancer cell uses in its metabolism. It has reportedly produced a regression rate of 20 percent in cancers of the cervix and respiratory tract.

Recommended Dosage

The usual dose of hexamethylmelamine for treating lung cancer is 400 to 500 milligrams per day, taken in three or four divided doses, between meals and at bedtime. This is continued for five days, followed by an interval of three weeks, after which the five-day course is repeated. For cancers of the reproductive tract, the recommended dosage is 400 to 500 milligrams per day for a course of twenty-one days each month.

Side Effects of Hexamethylmelamine

Initial side effects include nausea, vomiting, blood count changes (which are reversible), and rash—pruritus or eczema. However, following long-term use, numbness, tingling or prickling sensations, hallucinations, depression, confusion and drowsiness may be experienced. Peripheral neuropathy may continue after the drug has been discontinued.

Unless the benefits are greater than the risks, this drug

should not be taken by women of childbearing age. After taking this medication, patients should be monitored closely for changes in their white blood cell or platelet count.

IFOSFAMIDE

Tumors that respond to this anticancer drug include those of the ear, nose, throat, lung, testis, ovary, breast, uterus, kidney, pancreas, gastrointestinal tract, and bone. It has also been used to treat tumors of the lymphatic systems and soft tissue sarcoma tumors. Ifosfamide is frequently used with other anticancer drugs such as vincristine or methotrexate, and used in addition to radiation therapy.

How Ifosfamide Works

This drug works by damaging the DNA molecules of the cancer cells, thereby destroying them. These types of drugs are intended to work on the faster dividing cancer cells, but may also affect bone marrow cells and even the cells of the reproductive tract.

Recommended Dosage

Ifosfamide comes in dry powder vials of 500 milligrams, 1, and 2 grams. The drug is dissolved in water in a ratio of 1 gram per 12.5 milliliter of fluid, and further diluted in sodium chloride and dextrose solution of 4 percent (12 grams per 25 milliliters) for direct intravenous injection or slow infusion over a period of thirty minutes to two hours.

Usually a single daily dose over a period of three to ten days for a total of 8 to 10 grams per square meter of body surface is recommended.

Side Effects of Ifosfamide

Urinary tract disorders are common side effects of this drug. Confusion, lethargy, vomiting, nausea, temporary hair loss, restlessness, disorientation, mood changes, irritation of the mouth, diarrhea, nausea, changes in blood cell counts, and increased susceptibility to infections may occur during the course of treatment.

Women typically experience cessation of menstruation while taking ifosfamide, and men usually become temporarily sterile. It should not be taken by people who are allergic or sensitive to this or similar products such as cyclophosphamide. People who have serious kidney or liver impairment or urinary bladder bleeding should not use this drug.

INOSIPLEX (METHISOPRINOL)

Inosiplex is an antiviral drug, unique in that it not only fights the herpes zoster virus, but also it reinforces immune response to a disease called sclerosing panencephalitis, which impairs brain function and results in death within a year. This drug has also been used to treat Type A infectious hepatitis, cold sores and fever blisters, measles, and chicken pox.

How Inosiplex Works

Inosiplex combats viruses by encouraging the microbe-destroying action of elements of the blood called macrophages. It also stimulates the B and T lymphocytes, essential elements of the immune system that fight microorganisms such as viruses and fungi.

Recommended Dosage

This drug is available as 500 milligram tablets and as a syrup containing 5 grams per 100 milliliters or 8 grams per 120 milliliters. Adults initially take 100 milligrams per kilogram of body weight per day, after which a maintenance dose of 40 milligrams per kilogram of body weight per day is instituted. For children five and under, the initial dosage is the same as for adults, but the maintenance dose is 50 milligrams per kilogram of body weight per day. One teaspoonful of the syrup contains approximately 205 milligrams of inosiplex.

Side Effects of Inosiplex

Although it is usually a well-tolerated drug, it may cause nausea and vomiting when taken by mouth. People with gout must use caution with this drug since it increases uric acid levels.

INOSITOL NIACINATE (INOSITOL NICOTINATE)

Inositol niacinate is effective for relief of restless leg syndrome, cerebral arteriosclerosis, painful menstruation, cold hands and feet, chilblains, night cramps, Raynaud's phenomenon, intermittent claudication, Buerger's disease, acrocyanosis, erythrocyanosis, migraine, and cerebral arteriosclerosis. It can also assist in the treatment of hyperlipiproteinemia and hyperlipidemia, as well as necrobiosis lipoidica, a condition caused by atrophy of the skin.

How Inositol Niacinate Works

This drug increases blood circulation to arms and legs, so it is an effective therapy for conditions that are caused by poor circulation.

Recommended Dosage

The usual adult dosage of this medication is 400 to 500 milligrams three times daily, gradually increasing dosage to 4000 to 5000 milligrams. For night cramps and restless legs, people generally take 200 to 800 milligrams at night. To relieve the symptoms of cerebrovascular insufficiency, 1000 milligrams three times daily is the usual dosage.

Side Effects of Inositol Niacinate

The drug is generally well tolerated, with few side effects. These, however, may include nausea, vomiting, flushing, dizziness, blood pressure changes, and headache. This drug should not be used by people who are recovering from a stroke or heart attack.

LEVAMISOLE HYDROCHLORIDE

A strong weapon against intestinal worms, this drug has the added advantage of stimulating the body's immune system. This quality makes it a useful anticancer drug, especially against Hodgkin's disease. It is often used in conjunction with other anticancer drugs.

Levamisole hydrochloride is also of value in treating such autoimmune diseases as systemic lupus erythematosus, rheumatoid arthritis, herpes infections, leishmaniasis, warts, toxoplasmosis, aphthous ulcers of the mouth, and eosinophilia.

How Levamisole Hydrochloride Works

The Levamisole hydrochloride acts by paralyzing worms in the intestine. These worms are then discharged from the body during the elimination process. It appears to work as an immunostimulant by restoring depressed T-cell functions.

Recommended Dosage

This drug is available as 30, 50, and 150 milligram tablets and also as a syrup that provides 40 milligrams per teaspoonful of medication. The drug is usually administered as a single dose which may be repeated the following day. To treat roundworms, usually 150 milligrams per day for adults is given, and 3 milligrams per kilogram of body weight for children. For hookworms, the dose is 300 milligrams for adults and 8 milligrams per kilogram of body weight for children. When used to treat other conditions, dosages range from 50 to 1250 milligrams per day continuously or intermittently.

Side Effects of Levamisole Hydrochloride

Single doses have been reported to cause side effects ranging from insomnia, nausea and vomiting, nervousness, stomach ache or other gastric discomfort, as well as changes in sense of taste and smell. With long-term use, side effects include vasculitis (inflammation of the blood vessels), sensitivity to light, skin rash, and blood disorders.

LYMECYCLINE

This broad-spectrum antibiotic is effective against a variety of infections caused by various organisms. These include chronic bronchitis, genital infections, middle ear infections, sinusitis, severe acne, undulant fever, and trachoma.

How Lymecycline Works

Lymecycline resembles the well-known antibiotic tetracycline in its action, but is more efficiently absorbed when taken by mouth. Lymecycline in 150 milligram tablets is as powerful as 250 milligrams of tetracycline and is also more soluble. Because of this, smaller doses will work against a given infection. Lymecycline is thought to work by interfering with the ability of the bacteria to conduct their metabolic processes and build cell walls.

Recommended Dosage

The preferred adult dosage is 300 milligrams in the morning and again in the evening. If the infection is severe, the dosage may be increased to 1 to 2 grams daily.

Side Effects of Lymecycline

Reported side effects of this drug include nausea, vomiting, and diarrhea. These side effects may be milder than those of tetracycline. Care must be taken regarding the possibility of resistant strains of bacteria arising, resulting in suprainfections.

Like tetracycline, lymecycline can cause changes in the developing teeth of children and for this reason should not be used by them. Another side effect is discoloration of the fingernails. This drug is not recommended for people with impaired kidney function.

MECLOFENOXATE

This psychotropic drug is used to mitigate the effects of conditions such as stroke, mental retardation, alcoholism, drug abuse, senility, chemical poisoning, oxygen deprivation at birth or during surgery, cerebrovascular accidents, as well as visual impairment.

How Meclofenoxate Works

Meclofenoxate assists the brain in functioning more efficiently when it has a lowered supply of oxygen due to the above conditions. It boosts the metabolic rate and helps in performance of basic mental tasks, even when there is a deprivation of oxygen.

Recommended Dosage

This drug may be taken by mouth or by intravenous or intramuscular injection. The usual dose is two to six 500 milligram tablets every day.

Side Effects of Meclofenoxate

Drowsiness, depression, and motion sickness are commonly reported, in addition to overexcitability and insomnia. Those who are easily excitable, vulnerable to seizures, or who have severe high blood pressure probably should not take this medication.

METRONIDAZOLE PLUS NYSTATIN

This medication primarily treats trichomonas and monilia infections of the vaginal tract. While both drugs are available individually in the United States, this extremely effective combination product is only available outside the country.

How Metronidazole Plus Nystatin Works

Nystatin is an antifungal element, effective against candida albicans, which is responsible for moniliasis infections. Metronidazole works by being a direct trichomonacidal. It can actually wipe out 99 percent of the infecting organisms in a twenty-four-hour period.

Recommended Dosage

Metronidazole plus nystatin vaginal inserts each contain 500 milligrams of metronidazole and 100,000 units of nystatin. It is also supplied as vaginal inserts of 100,000 units of nystatin plus 200 milligrams metronidazole tablets. Vaginal inserts and creams are used for ten days.

If the infection persists, a second ten-day course of treatment is recommended. It is important that sexual partners and contacts also begin this medication, because an untreated person can reinfect the treated partner.

Side Effects of Metronidazole Plus Nystatin

Common side effects include vaginal burning and a bad taste in the mouth. Infrequent side effects include nervous system disorders, such as ataxia and loss of motor coordination.

People who have experienced neurological disorders, blood diseases, hypothyroidism, or hypoadrenalism should avoid this product. Those who take this drug should not use alcoholic beverages during the course of treatment, as alcohol may result in nausea and diarrhea.

PIRAGLUTARGINE (ARGININE PIDOLATE, ARGININE PYROGLUTAMATE)

This controversial drug is believed to stimulate more efficient brain function among the mentally retarded and those afflicted with senility. Piraglutargine's effectiveness is based on the theory that glutamate, which composes a great deal of the brain's tissue, deteriorates with age and can be replaced.

How Piraglutargine Works

Piraglutargine is a glutamate, which is thought to encourage brain function, thus allowing for more efficient information processing and memory enhancement.

Recommended Dosage

The recommended dosage is 500 milligrams to 1000 milligrams per day.

Side Effects of Piraglutargine

This is a natural product, which is present in many common foods. No adverse effects have been recorded as of this writing.

PIZOTYLINE MALEATE (PIZOTIFEN MALEATE)

This drug is used to alleviate the pain of migraine headaches, to treat depression, encourage appetite, and resolve pruritus, carcinoid syndrome, and carotodynia. It is also used for Cushing's disease, a disorder of the adrenal gland that manifests in weakness and loss of protein.

How Pizotyline Maleate Works

Serotonin is a nervous system chemical that affects many functions. Pizotyline actually blocks serotonin and prevents some unwanted impulses from being conducted across nervous system tissue.

Recommended Dosage

The usual recommended dosage is 1 to 5 milligrams daily. The most common dosage is 500 micrograms in the morning, and 1 milligram at bedtime. To treat severe conditions, intake has been raised as high as 3 to 8 milligrams daily. The drug is not advised for children.

Side Effects of Pizotyline Maleate

The most common side effect is stimulated appetite with concomitant weight gain. More infrequent side effects include impotence, confusion, nausea, muscle pain, headache, edema, and dry mouth. Pizotyline maleate may cause drowsiness and should not be used when driving or operating machinery. It also interacts with alcohol, hypnotics, sedatives, and psychotropic medications.

Some may develop a tolerance to this medication. People who are taking monomamine oxidase inhibitors should not take this drug, nor should those with ulcers or obstructions of the pyloroduodenal area. Those with heart disease, diabetes, glaucoma, enlarged prostate, or impaired liver or kidney function should use this drug with caution.

PYRITINOL HYDROCHLORIDE
(PYRITHIOXINE HYDROCHLORIDE)

This drug is used to alleviate symptoms of stroke, senile dementia, brain injury, mental retardation, headache, speech disorders, cerebral arteriosclerosis, apathy, and other disorders that occur when blood flow to the brain is reduced.

How Pyritinol Hydrochloride Works

Pyritinol hydrochloride stimulates brain function and efficiency by chemically increasing the amount of blood sugar that reaches the brain.

Recommended Dosage

The usual dosage is one 100 milligram tablet or one teaspoonful of syrup containing 200 milligrams per 5 milliliters of medication three times a day. Pyritinol hydrochloride can also be administered intravenously in doses of 200 to 400 milligrams daily.

Side Effects of Pyritinol Hydrochloride

Pyritinol hydrochloride has been reported to bring on nausea, gastrointestinal discomfort, dizziness, and headache.

RAUBASINE (AJMALICINE)

Raubasine is used to treat many conditions including migraine, cerebral ischemia, headaches due to head injuries, Buerger's disease, reduced flow of blood to the arms and legs, cold feet and hands, blood vessel disorders associated with diabetes, lesions on the hands and feet due to poor circulation, Raynaud's phenomenon, night cramps, high blood pressure, both essential and secondary pre-eclampsia and eclampsia, acrocyanosis, and coronary artery insufficiency.

How Raubasine Works

Raubasine is derived from the rose periwinkle plant, and has a tranquilizing effect much like reserpine.

Recommended Dosage

Raubasine is available as 1 and 5 milligram tablets. The usual dosage is 1 or 2 milligrams three times daily before meals, when taken continuously, or 5 milligrams two or three times per day before meals, on alternate weeks.

Side Effects of Raubasine

The side effects of raubasine resemble those of reserpine, including difficulty in breathing, skin rash, nausea, diarrhea, and dizziness. People who have bronchial asthma, gall bladder disorder, epilepsy, heart disease, or suffer from stomach or duodenal ulcers, ulcerative colitis, or mental depression should not take this drug.

RAZOXANE

This is an anticancer drug that is often employed when alternative methods of therapy have become necessary. Razoxane is active against leukemia, lymphatic cancers, and solid tumors and is used by itself or as an adjunct to other therapies. Razoxane has also been effective in treating nonmalignant skin disorders such as psoriasis.

How Razoxane Works

Razoxane interferes with the multiplication process of the cancer cells. It also seems to increase the impact of radiation therapy, making it more destructive to the cancer cells.

Recommended Dosage

Since dosages vary greatly according to the type of tumor being treated, consult a physician.

Side Effects of Razoxane

Just as with many forms of chemotherapy, razoxane may cause loss of hair, nausea, vomiting, diarrhea, and changes in skin color. People who have had chemotherapy before taking razoxane may experience a rise in white blood cells and an abnormal decrease in blood platelets.

TENIPOSIDE

This is an anticancer drug used to treat tumors of the lymphatic system or lymphomas, particularly in Hodgkin's disease. It is also used to treat solid tumors, such as tumors of the brain and the bladder.

How Teniposide Works

Teniposide is chemically related to etoposide, another cancer-fighting drug. Both drugs act by interfering with the cancer cell's ability to divide. Teniposide is extracted from the mayapple or American mandrake root.

Recommended Dosage

This medication is available as injection ampules containing 50 milligrams per 5 milliliters of medication. Usually, dosage is determined according to the standard of 30 milligrams per square meter of body surface area for five days.

Malignant lymphomas and brain tumors have been treated with dosages as high as 40 to 50 milligrams per square meter of body surface. The drug is given in five-day courses, with an interval of five to fifteen days between. In order to gain remission, four or five cycles of treatment may be needed.

Side Effects of Teniposide

This is a highly toxic anticancer drug that can cause hair loss, nausea, vomiting, reduction in white cell and platelet count, and other side effects common to chemotherapy drugs. A side effect of the injection may be a sudden drop in blood pressure, and the patient may notice inflammation at the site of the injection.

People may experience lowered resistance to some infections during a course of chemotherapy, and this drug may affect production of sperm or ova. Those with blood disorders or who are currently fighting bacterial infections may experience complications, as can those with impaired kidney or liver function, and neurologic or cardiovascular disorders.

TETRABENAZINE

Tetrabenazine acts against nervous system and muscle disorders such as tardive dyskinesia, Huntington's chorea, senile chorea, involuntary twitchings, and tics of the muscles of the mouth, hands, and fingers.

How Tetrabenazine Works

Tetrabenazine stops unwanted muscle movements by interrupting the transmission of impulses to muscles. It affects the storage of the naturally occurring chemicals that assist in that transmission, keeping the signals from getting through to the affected area and preventing the involuntary movement.

Recommended Dosage

The initial adult dosage of tetrabenazine is one 25 milligram tablet twice daily, followed by gradual 25 milligram increases every day for three or four days until the desired effect is obtained.

Side Effects of Tetrabenazine

There has been evidence in the laboratory that higher doses of this drug can cause breast enlargement. Reports of side effects include choking attacks, difficulty in swallowing, as well as parkinsonism symptoms and drowsiness, blood pressure changes, anxiety, restlessness, and slowed heartbeat.

Tetrabenazine may aggravate the manifestations of parkinsonism or depression. Since this drug is manufactured with tartrazine, an artificial food coloring, people who have an allergy to that chemical should avoid it.

Using Tetrabenazine in Combination with Other Drugs

Tetrabenazine interferes with the action of levodopa and reserpine. In addition, this drug interacts with alcohol, monoamine oxidase inhibitors, antidepressants, and high blood pressure medications.

TREOSULFAN

The primary use for this drug is in treating ovarian cancer. It is usually combined with other treatments. Because treosulfan is toxic to many cells throughout the body, including bone marrow cells, it is expected that white blood cell and platelet counts will be lowered during a cycle of treatment. Within a month or so of discontinuing treatment, the cell counts generally return to normal.

How Treosulfan Works

This drug is an alkylating agent that achieves its therapeutic effect by interfering with the DNA of the cancer cell, making the cancer incapable of reproducing and spreading. Because it interferes with cell division, this drug can also influence normal cells, and since it is used in the reproductive area, a woman usually becomes sterile while taking this course of medication. Most of the time, the sterility is reversible, but not always.

Recommended Dosage

This medication is available as 25 milligram capsules and as a powder that can be injected after mixing with fluid. The common oral dose is 1 gram or four capsules daily in four divided doses for one month, followed by one month without treatment. After this, blood cell counts are taken, and the treatment may be adjusted on the basis of the results. The treatment cycle is then repeated.

If radiation is also used in conjunction with treosulfan, only half the usual dosage is generally used. The intravenous dosage is 5 to 15 grams every one to three weeks. A maintenance dose may also be used depending on how low the white cell count falls.

Side Effects of Treosulfan

Like other anticancer drugs, treosulfan has the side effects of hair loss, nausea, vomiting, and skin eruptions. Since this drug is so caustic, care must be exercised in handling the capsule as the substance can cause irritation and inflammation.

TRILOSTANE

This drug is active against an adrenal disorder that is caused by overproduction of hormones, as well as Cushing's syndrome.

How Trilostane Works

Trilostane affects the adrenal gland, lowering the amount of chemical that causes disorders such as Cushing's syndrome.

Recommended Dosage

Trilostane may be taken by mouth. It is available as 60 milligram capsules, and the usual range of dosage is 120 to 480 milligrams per day in divided doses. The maximum recommended daily dosage is 960 milligrams per day.

Side Effects of Trilostane

At higher doses, nausea, runny nose, vomiting, flushing, and edema of the palate may take place. It is important that blood tests be taken throughout treatment to monitor the levels of hormone. This drug may influence the potassium levels in the blood and may interact with diuretics, as well as the effectiveness of oral contraceptives. People with impaired kidney or liver functions need to use great caution when taking this drug.

TROXERUTIN (VITAMIN P4)

This medication is used to alleviate disorders of the vascular system, including varicose veins, diabetic retinopathy, heavy or swollen legs, burning or tingling sensations (paresthesias), hemorrhoids, water retention in the ankles, night cramps, poor limb circulation during pregnancy, superficial thrombophlebitis, restless legs, Raynaud's phenomenon, ulcers, and skin inflammation that comes with insufficient flow of blood.

How Troxerutin Works

Troxerutin is composed of an element found in common buckwheat. It is thought to strengthen the capillaries and smaller veins of the vascular system. Thus, it allows more oxygen-carrying blood to reach the tissues and also to increase the volume of lymph making its way through the body.

Recommended Dosage

Oral troxerutin should be taken at mealtime. This drug may also be applied as an ointment. The usual oral dosage is two 100 milligram tablets or one 200 or 300 milligram capsule three times a day for up to four weeks at first. This course is followed by a maintenance dosage at lower levels.

Side Effects of Troxerutin

Stomach upset or other gastrointestinal discomfort, headaches, and flushing may be experienced. This drug should not be taken during pregnancy.

VINCAMINE

Such conditions as stroke, lack of oxygen to the brain, and other cerebral conditions can be treated with vincamine, which can also help relieve psychiatric conditions that afflict the elderly.

How Vincamine Works

Vincamine works by increasing the circulation of blood in the brain and helping it to use oxygen more effectively, thus allowing for better mental functioning.

Recommended Dosage

Vincamine can be given in an intravenous or intramuscular injection, or by mouth in 40 to 80 milligram dosages.

Side Effects of Vincamine

People with hypertension or cardiac impairment should use this drug with great caution. It may also cause stomach discomfort.

VINDESINE SULFATE

This is a drug that assists in the chemotherapeutic treatment of certain types of cancers, such as childhood leukemia, malignant melanoma, and bone marrow cancers of older people. It is also employed in treating cancers that have been resistant to other forms of therapy or to treat relapses.

How Vindesine Sulfate Works

Vindesine sulfate works by interfering with the process of reproduction in the cancer cells. It is manufactured by a process that uses the periwinkle plant and is stronger than vincristine sulfate or vinblastine sulfate.

Recommended Dosage

This drug is injected into a large vein, along with a drug called hyaluronidase, to reduce irritation of surrounding tissues.

For adults, the usual dose is 3 to 4 milligrams per square meter of body area; and 4 to 5 milligrams per square meter of body area for children. The drug is given in one injection and repeated every week. This drug should be administered only in a hospital under the guidance of a specialist in treating cancer. Changes in blood count can mandate changes in the dosage.

Side Effects of Vindesine Sulfate

The usual side effects of hair loss, nausea, vomiting, and inflammation of the tongue and mouth may occur, and, infrequently, convulsions. People suffering from bacterial infections should not take this drug, nor should pregnant women or nursing mothers, since it is so toxic and causes changes in reproductive cells that may result in birth defects. People whose white blood cell or platelet count is down following other chemotherapies may not be candidates for this drug.

CHAPTER X

AIDS and AIDS Drugs

My rationale for including a separate chapter on AIDS and AIDS drugs is threefold. First, it took the onset of the AIDS crisis to bring the problems involving the FDA approval process to light. And without the protests and the pressures of the AIDS activist groups, there would have been no change in the FDA policy regarding mail-order importation of drugs from foreign countries.

Second, AIDS activist groups were among the first to make *widespread public use* of the mail to import medically significant treatments for their disease. Long before the FDA officially changed its policy, AIDS patients had banded together to bring foreign pharmaceuticals into the US by mail. In fact, one HIV-positive person that I talked to said the idea was really old hat to him. He started importing megadoses of quality vitamins from Switzerland and herbs from the Orient as soon as he learned he was HIV positive.

Third, it is estimated that there are nearly 800,000 HIV-positive people alive who have not yet developed AIDS or AIDS Related Complex (ARC) symptoms. Many of these people live in places where they do not have access to the appropriate information and treatments that are needed to lengthen their lives. This chapter is intended to be of help to these individuals.

WHAT IS AIDS?

AIDS is the most serious manifestation of HIV infections, a disease which is caused by a single virus. This virus has been identified under different names throughout the years, but is now called HIV or human immunodeficiency virus. It acts by attacking specific cells in the body's immune system, rendering the body unable to defend itself against a variety of infections and illnesses. It is not the virus specifically that kills the affected person; the infections and illnesses that result from the body's inability to marshall its own defenses gradually weaken the body to the point of death.

Even the healthy body is constantly being invaded by microorganisms capable of causing infection, but we are unaware that our immune system is able to repel most of these invaders. This is why healthy people stay healthy. When our immune system is unable to deter an infection, such as an attack of influenza, we become ill.

HOW HIV INFECTION LEADS TO AIDS

The main element of the body's immune system that is attacked by HIV is called the T4 or "helper" cell. These cells activate the body's entire immune system to protect against invading bacteria and viruses. Without a high T4 helper cell count in the bloodstream, the body's immune system cannot function properly and resist disease. Thus the body becomes susceptible to all manner of diseases, the most common of which are infections, tumors, and cancers.

HIV actually invades and takes over the T4 helper cell. This infected cell then starts to produce more of the virus. Then these new viruses spread into the bloodstream and attack other cells. The infected T4 helper cells thus become an enemy of the body, rather than a defense.

Once HIV becomes entrenched, infected cells attach

themselves to other infected T4 helper cells to become virtual clumps of virus-producing cells. Infected cells are also able to chemically fool healthy T4 helper cells into attacking other healthy cells. The result is that the immune system begins to self-destruct by sending out antibodies to attack healthy cells.

Over time, the number of T4 helper cells declines. Despite the body's attempts to replace T4 cells, they die off faster than they can be produced. The lower the number of T4 helper cells, the higher the likelihood of the body falling victim to infections and illnesses. Without treatment, symptoms of ARC begin to occur. As the infection spreads, a full-blown AIDS condition develops.

Project Inform, a nonprofit organization in San Francisco, offers these statistics. Infected people lose about 10 to 15 percent of their total T cells each year. In untreated cases, HIV leads to AIDS or ARC in seven years for 78 percent of the cases. Children born with HIV and people infected by blood transfusion get sick more quickly. No group has shown the ability to develop immunity to the virus.

TREATMENT OF AIDS

The prevailing philosophy of HIV treatment today, is that the disease must be treated as early as possible, long before it reaches the stage of life-threatening AIDS from which there is no known recovery. The first step in preventing AIDS is to take an HIV antibody test. Once an individual has a positive HIV antibody test, treatments are available which can slow the spread of the virus. Most treatments are aimed at preventing or lessening the severity of infections and illnesses that people get once the immune system is weakened by HIV.

It was exactly this argument that was used to force the FDA to speed up its approval of AZT, the first AIDS drug to receive such approval. But it is sad to note that even in 1990, with an FDA-approved drug on the market, relatively few of the people at risk are tested as quickly as they should be.

On top of this problem there is a secondary problem. Many people delay treatment once they find out that they have tested HIV positive, since initially they do not show any symptoms of the AIDS. However, whether they are symptom free or not, the infection progresses inevitably. In fact, by the time symptoms begin, severe damage to the individual's immune system is likely to have already occurred.

Managing HIV infection usually involves three types of treatment. First antiviral drugs are begun to slow down the rate at which HIV reproduces. Secondarily, drugs called immunomodulators are used to bolster the body's own immune system. The third method of treatment against HIV consists of preventive measures against infections due to an already weakened immune system. These drugs, called OI preventatives, are administered typically when the T4 helper cell count drops dangerously low. This triple-pronged attack is the best means available today to help people survive HIV infection.

Most physicians now believe that treatment with antiviral drugs should begin as soon as a person tests positive for HIV. (Recent studies have shown that in most cases early treatment with AZT greatly slows the progression to AIDS.) Even though there is no evidence of AIDS or any other symptoms, the disease relentlessly progresses in its destruction of the body's immune system. The goal is to slow the progression of HIV before it gains a foothold and the T4 helper cell count begins to fall.

Researchers believe that the best time to start treatment is when the T4 helper count is still above 500. When the count is high, there are enough T cells functioning to trigger an effective immune response to fight off infection. When the count falls too low, it is very difficult to rebuild. Counts below 200 indicate that a person is at very great risk of opportunistic infections such as *Pneumocystis carinii* pneumonia (PCP), the virulent lung infection that often kills or seriously weakens many AIDS patients.

HOW TO FIND OUT MORE ABOUT AIDS AND AIDS TREATMENTS

Project Inform provides all the latest AIDS treatment information toll free at 1-800-334-7422 in California; 1-800-822-7422 nationally; or locally at 1-415-558-8669. The *AIDS Treatment News*, reports on more experimental treatments. For information, call 1-415-255-0588 or write Box 411256, San Francisco, CA 94141. Also check *Treatment Issues* which is available from GMHC, Dept. of Medical Information, 129 W. 20 Street, New York, NY 10011.

DRUGS USED IN THE TREATMENT OF AIDS

As of mid 1990 there are more than seventy drugs in development for the treatment of AIDS or ARC. Most of these fall into five general classes: antivirals that slow or prevent the virus from multiplying; immunomodulators that boost the immune system; anti-infectives that fight AIDS-related bacterial and fungal infections; vaccines that prevent infection; and cytokines that regulate the growth of cells and counter some of the toxic effects of other drugs.

Drugs that have been approved by the FDA for the treatment of AIDS or ARC include: Retrovir (AZT), Septra (a PCP treatment), NebuPent (aerosol pentamidine for PCP prevention), Cytovene (ganciclover for the treatment of cytomegalovirus retinitis), and Diflucan (fluconazole for the treatment of cryptococcal meningitis). All other drugs for the treatment of AIDS or ARC that are discussed here and elsewhere have yet to be approved. Their use is sure to pose many unknown risks.

The following is a selected listing of medications that are currently being used in the AIDS underground for treating various conditions related to HIV infection, as well as information about their availability, action, and proper usage. These drugs are available outside the United States by mail order. For those drugs that are widely available in the US, foreign prices are generally much lower. Please note that some of these drugs are not listed in the sample price lists at the end of Appendix I. Interested readers should contact some of the listed suppliers at the beginning of Appendix I to check availability.

ACYCLOVIR

Acyclovir (ACV) is an antiviral that it is widely used to treat the herpes simplex infection. Recently, it has begun to be used by people with ARC and AIDS. It is frequently prescribed for people with HIV-related infections, including shingles, hairy leukoplakia, cytomegalovirus, and Epstein-Barr virus. Many researchers feel that these types of infections help activate the underlying HIV infection. Thus, using acyclovir to treat those infections may potentially reduce the progression of the HIV infection.

There has also been speculation that acyclovir can actually be useful in the treatment of HIV itself, perhaps by strengthening the body's immune response to AZT, or diminishing the side effects of AZT. Because of this, acyclovir is often prescribed along with AZT.

How Acyclovir Works

In high concentrations, acyclovir limits reproduction of HIV in lab cultures. However, this has not been confirmed in human studies. There is evidence that acyclovir works to heighten the effects of AZT and lower the incidence of opportunistic infections. The result of this is that AZT may then be taken at lower dosages.

Recent studies have shown that acyclovir is not effective against the primary HIV infection itself, nor can it reduce the side effects of AZT. But reports from patients and physicians using acyclovir are generally positive, in that the drug is useful in controlling the manifestations of HIV infection, especially when used in combination with other drugs.

Recommended Dosage

Many physicians suggest the following dosages when using acyclovir in HIV-related infections:

For hairy leukoplakia, high doses are required, from 1800 to 3000 milligrams per day when lesions are present. When the lesions shrink or disappear, dosages can be reduced to 1200 milligrams per day for long-term therapy.

For shingles, moderate to high doses are required, depending on the severity. This means a dose ranging from 1200 milligrams to as high as 2400 milligrams per day until the problem has cleared for several days.

For cytomegalovirus-related skin infections (CMV), the dosage varies from 2400 milligrams to more than 4000 milligrams per day, since acyclovir is only moderately effective against CMV.

Side Effects of Acyclovir

Standard dosages of acyclovir seldom produce severe side effects. However, at higher doses short-term side effects may include nausea, vomiting, headaches, diarrhea, dizziness, anorexia, fatigue, and muscle cramps.

Long-term high dose users sometimes report tingling in the fingers and toes.

Using Acyclovir in Combination with Other Drugs

The most effective combination seems to be a mix of low dose AZT, full dose dextran sulfate, and a moderate to high dose of acyclovir. Good results have also been reported when using dextran sulfate with acyclovir or ribavirin with acyclovir.

AZT

AZT is probably the best known of all the AIDS drugs, and one of the few which has FDA approval for treatment of HIV infection. AZT was developed in the 1960s as a cancer treatment, for which it proved largely ineffective. In 1984, the Center for Disease Control in Atlanta declared AZT as a drug that was active against human immunodeficiency virus in the body. The FDA finally approved AZT as a treatment for early stage HIV infection in February 1990.

How AZT Works

AZT works by inhibiting reverse transcriptase, an enzyme which is essential to production of the HIV virus. AZT does this by providing a substitute for one of the proteins which the HIV virus seeks out to join as part of its reproductive cycle. When the HIV virus joins with the AZT-produced lookalike, the reproductive cycle of the virus is broken. Because of its action, AZT appears to slow or prevent production of new virus; unfortunately, it has no action against cells that are already infected.

Recommended Dosage

Research seems to indicate that there is not an ideal dosage for AZT. The newest available data lead to a dosage recommendation of 300 milligrams per day. (Note: the FDA still recommends 600 milligrams per day.) AZT is usually taken every four hours on a very regular schedule because it breaks down rapidly in the body. Many people set an alarm for nighttime administration, though some physicians say this is not necessary, suggesting instead that patients take acetaminophen with AZT at bedtime in hopes of extending the drug's half life.

Side Effects of AZT

The down side of AZT is its well-known side effects. In the first major study, 31 percent of those on 1200 milligrams per day dosage of AZT required blood transfusions to combat the anemia which developed due to the toxicity of the drug and its destructive action on the red blood cell–producing bone marrow. Many of these individuals required multiple transfusions. It is now generally recognized that such side effects do not justify whatever benefit might be gained from this high dosage.

Other side effects include headache, nausea, hypertension, and a general feeling of malaise or illness. These problems usually subside within a few weeks, if the patient continues to take the drug and tolerate the side effects.

Using AZT in Combination with Other Drugs

AZT is often used in combination with other drugs such as acyclovir. Acyclovir is used in doses ranging from 1200 to 2000 milligrams daily. The combination of AZT and acyclovir can limit the outbreak of herpes, control hairy leukoplatia, and reduce complications of cyto-megalovirus.

AZT is also sometimes used in combination with dex-tran sulfate, DTC or disulfiram, and acyclovir.

COMPOUND Q

Compound Q comes from the root tubers of a Chinese plant called Trichosanthes kirilowii. It belongs to a new class of antiviral drugs called cytotoxis or antiviral plant proteins. These differ in action from the current antivirals such as AZT, which work by inhibiting reproduction of the virus.

Antiviral proteins such as Compound Q actually poison only those cells which are in some way infected or dam-aged by a virus. Thus, in theory they could destroy the HIV-infected cells, leaving the others intact and free from infection.

Informal reports as of June 1990 suggest that there is strong evidence to suggest that Compound Q will turn out to be an extremely effective AIDS treatment that serves to increase the number of T4 helper cells. However, for-mal studies have yet to be reported. So caution is called for.

How Compound Q Works

Compound Q works by attacking and destroying cells which are infected with HIV. Healthy cells are not affected by Compound Q. This drug is most effective on people with an infection that is not well established, but it also helps those at later stages of the HIV infection and with AIDS.

Underground reports of results from treatment pro-grams indicate benefit for many patients after using Compound Q just three times. The drug appears to be dangerous for people with T4 counts below 50 or 100, especially if there is evidence of HIV in the brain or nervous system.

Recommended Dosage

Call Project Inform for the latest recommendation.

Side Effects of Compound Q

Side effects include mild fevers lasting for up to two to five days, muscle aches and pains, mental disorganization, joint pain and swelling, various rashes, and some hives. However, most side effects are not serious enough to stop drug use.

ddC (DIDEOXYCYTIDINE)

ddC is an antiviral drug that is an alternative to AZT and ddI. Hoffmann-LaRoche, the drug's manufacturer, is now beginning to make it available to small numbers of people who either do not benefit from or cannot tolerate AZT and ddI.

This antiviral has been around for more than three years, but early high dosages led to severe side effects in the form of sometimes irreversible tingling and numbness in the hands and feet. However, recent studies have shown that low dosages (one-sixth the original level) are effective and have a much lower incidence rate of neuropathy.

How ddC Works

Like ddI and AZT, ddC works by preventing HIV from reproducing. It does not stop or eliminate the HIV infection, but it slows the damage.

Recommended Dosage

The current recommended dose of ddC is 2 milligrams per day.

Side Effects of ddC

The major side effect of ddC is the painful peripheral neuropathy that occurs in about 10 percent of the people using it.

Using ddC in Combination with Other Drugs

There are underground (unofficial) reports that have leaked from two formal studies currently underway that ddC used in conjunction with low dosages of AZT has led to some of the best results ever to be found with antivirals.

ddI (DIDEOXYINOSINE)

ddI is an antiviral drug that was originally developed by the National Cancer Institute as an alternative to AZT. The pharmaceutical firm of Bristol-Myers holds a government license to market this drug, and due to positive results from early testing, they have made ddI available to those who can not tolerate AZT.

Although further research of ddI's effectiveness is needed, initial response to ddI suggests that it may come to replace AZT as the treatment of choice for AIDS. For example, two recent studies (reported in May 1990) have shown that ddI offers real hope for HIV-infected people. Both studies showed that low doses of ddI given once or twice a day resulted in a significant increase in the number of T4 helper cells and a reduction in the amount of AIDS virus present. Patients also reported more energy and less fatigue after only six weeks of use. Unlike AZT, the use of ddI did not lead to anemia.

How ddI Works

Like AZT, ddI works by preventing HIV from reproducing. It does not stop or eliminate the HIV infection, but it is capable of slowing the damage caused to the immune system by the virus.

Recommended Dosage

ddI is much easier to use than AZT because it does not break down as quickly in the blood as AZT. ddI is usually taken once or twice daily in a very low dosage. (Call Project Inform to obtain the most current recommendation.)

Side Effects of ddI

The reported side effects of ddI include headache, insomnia, and increased uric acid levels. Peripheral neuropathy has also been reported. However, this is reversible when detected early and once ddI is discontinued.

The real concern for ddI users is the recent discovery of pancreatitis as a possible side effect. In the first few months of 1990 there have been five cases of death by pancreatitis that have also been reported by ddI users.

Using ddI in Combination with Other Drugs

It is hoped that using ddI in conjunction with AZT, or on alternating days, might reduce the toxic side effects of AZT and minimize the development of drug resistance. There is no information available on how ddI interacts with other commonly used AIDS drugs such as acyclovir.

DEXTRAN SULFATE

Dextran sulfate is an antiviral which is believed to work against the HIV infection. It was first produced in the 1950s and has been used in Japan and elsewhere for years to help lower blood cholesterol and as a blood thinner (anticoagulant). Some forms of dextran sulfate are sold over the counter in Japan, and some forms are used along with blood transfusions to reduce the chance of blood clots.

How Dextran Sulfate Works

Dextran sulfate inhibits production of reverse transcriptase, which is a protein required by the HIV virus to reproduce. This effect is similar to the way AZT produces a decoy copy of the necessary protein, which the virus mistakenly uses and is then unable to replicate itself. Thus, the virus in the blood cannot attack new T4 helper cells. But the already infected cells remain active, and these may attack the uninfected cells by linking up with them.

There are conflicting opinions as to dextran sulfate's ability to cross the blood-brain barrier and hit the HIV infection attacking the brain and spinal fluid. Because of the large size of the dextran sulfate molecule, it is believed that this drug is incapable of diffusing across the blood-brain barrier.

Dextran sulfate first gained recognition in 1987, with an article in the *Lancet*, the British journal of medicine. Researchers reported that the drug had effectiveness at levels tolerable in the human body against the infection and destruction of T4 helper cell cultures under attack by HIV. A second report suggested that the compound increased the strength of AZT in certain proportions.

232

Recommended Dosage

Current studies of dextran sulfate are using from 2700 to 5400 milligrams per day. The drug is supplied in 300 milligram tablets; usually two or three tablets are taken at once, about six hours apart, resulting in a total daily intake of nine or more pills.

Side Effects of Dextran Sulfate

Diarrhea that is only partially managed by antidiarrhea medication seems to be the worst side effect. Other common side effects are those associated with anticoagulants. Dextran sulfate may cause slow healing of wounds, making it unsuitable for people with hemophilia or other blood disorders. There have been some reports of insomnia and slightly raised liver toxicity. These side effects seem to increase over time. People who have low blood platelet counts are probably not good candidates for dextran sulfate.

Using Dextran Sulfate in Combination with Other Drugs

A small number of physicians are presently using dextran sulfate from Japan in combination with AZT, acyclovir, AL721, or other available treatments. These physicians have reported increased T4 helper cell counts after nine to twelve weeks. However, two physicians concluded that dosages under 1800 milligrams per day are not effective.

DTC

DTC is available in France under the name of Imuthiol and can be purchased as a raw chemical in the US. DTC is thought to have both immune boosting and antiviral capabilities.

Preliminary research indicates that DTC increases T4 helper cell count in some patients. However, this action tends to plateau over time, stopping totally after a number of months. DTC works best on patients with a reasonably high T4 helper cell count and does little for those with low cell counts.

How DTC Works

DTC activates the body's liver to manufacture hepatosin. This hormone is thought to help T4 helper cells mature and function to ward off the HIV infection.

Recommended Dosage

DTC is taken rectally, by dissolving it in water (about 10 cc). Dosage for DTC ranges between 600 and 800 milligrams, depending on body weight.

Due to the difficulty in obtaining and using DTC, many physicians recommend Antabuse, which is often prescribed for alcoholism treatment. Antabuse decomposes in the body to become DTC, so it is thought to have the same effects.

Side Effects of DTC

Common side effects include nausea and stomach cramps along with a poor interactive effect for those who use alcohol.

FLUCONAZOLE

Fluconazole is an antifungal agent that was originally developed in England by Pfizer for the treatment of vaginal yeast infections. It has recently (May 1990) been recommended by the National Institute of Allergy and Infectious Diseases as a maintenance therapy against cryptococcal meningitis and other fungal infections for people with AIDS.

How Fluconazole Works

Fluconazole works by inhibiting ergosterol, which is essential to the integrity and functioning of the fungal cell membrane.

Recommended Dosage

The recommended dosage is 400 milligrams the first day followed by 200 milligrams per day until at least ten days after testing negative for the meningitis. Lifetime maintenance therapy is recommended by many experts.

Side Effects of Fluconazole

Research suggests that fluconazole has fewer side effects than amphotericin B, which had been the previous treatment of choice. Reported side effects include skin rash, nausea, and rare instances of liver damage.

NALTREXONE

Naltrexone has been used in the past to treat heroin and other opiate addictions. It belongs to a class of drugs known as narcotic antagonists which work by interfering with the body's usual response to opiate drugs. The interesting aspect of naltrexone has to do with its ability to influence some aspects of the body's immune system.

How Naltrexone Works

Naltrexone stimulates the body's production of endorphins, natural substances that help to regulate the function of the nervous system. Opiate drugs imitate the effect of endorphins, which have been called the body's natural pain killers. A high dosage of opiate actually exceeds the body's natural endorphin level and creates a feeling of euphoria or well-being. When this occurs, the body shuts down its production of natural endorphins. Naltrexone, by stimulating the production of endorphins, blocks the reception of opiates.

Endorphins also link the immune system and the central nervous system. White blood cells attract endorphins, because they have receptor sites which are similar to the opiate receptors on nerve cells.

Some researchers believe that the HIV infection works to lower endorphin levels and to decrease the sensitivity of the receptor sites. AIDS patients also show high levels of alpha interferon, which is another endorphinlike chemical. This high level of alpha interferon is thought to signal the brain to lower its production of endorphins, thus further disturbing the immune response of the body.

Small amounts of naltrexone are thought to reestablish the normal regulation of immune functions by increasing endorphin levels; naltrexone also seems to reduce high levels of alpha interferon in the blood as well.

In limited studies it has been shown that naltrexone improves the immune response for those taking it, when compared to a control group. However, improvement was only noted for those patients who, on the basis of alpha-interferon testing, are classified as responders to naltrexone therapy.

Recommended Dosage

The recommended dosage for HIV is 2.75 milligrams per day. It is supplied in tablets. The liquid form is prepared by grinding two 50 milligram tablets and mixing their granules into 100 milliliters of a neutral fluid. The liquid is drawn up into a dropper until 2.75 milliliters is dispensed. The liquid may then be squirted directly into the mouth.

Side Effects of Naltrexone

No side effects have been reported.

Using Naltrexone in Combination with Other Drugs

If you are currently using naltrexone for drug-abuse therapy, you cannot use it for HIV therapy. The dosage for addiction treatment is too high to be of proper use in HIV infection therapy as an immunomodulator.

Some who have used naltrexone along with AZT report an increased immune response, although that may be due to the effects of AZT alone.

PENTAMADINE

One of the most serious manifestations of the HIV infection as it progresses to AIDS is *Pneumocystis carinii* pneumonia (PCP), a potentially lethal lung infection caused by the pneumocystis protozoa. Although this organism causes PCP in HIV infected individuals, it is harmless to people with healthy immune systems. In fact, some researchers believe that the organism lies dormant in most people and HIV reactivates it.

PCP was comparatively rare until the spread of HIV infection. It begins with nonspecific symptoms including fever, fatigue, and weight loss. These symptoms usually occur prior to any respiratory difficulties. Over time the patient develops a serious cough, accompanied by fever and wheezing. Although most people come through their first bout of PCP, it often returns and increases in severity.

How Pentamadine Works

Once a patient is hospitalized with PCP, treatment usually begins with the oral administration of common antibiotics such as Septra (also known as Bactrim or trimethoprim-sulfamethoxazole). Adverse side effects are very common on these drugs. If the patient doesn't show improvement, pentamidine is administered intravenously. Pentamidine is also an antibiotic that has been used since the 1940s for protozoal infections.

Recommended Dosage

New studies have demonstrated that pentamidine, administered in an inhaler mist form, is the most effective way to allow therapeutic concentrations of pentamidine to reach the lungs, without actually circulating in the rest of the body at such high levels.

Ideal aerosol pentamidine dosage is under study, with amounts tested ranging from 30 milligrams twice monthly to 300 milligrams twice monthly.

After a vial of pentamidine has been opened, the solution is mixed with sterile water. The drug is good for only twenty-four hours after opening, and it is best to discard unused amounts.

Side Effects of Pentamidine

The most common side effect reported with aerosol pentamidine is a cough or dry, raspy throat, which can be minimized or eliminated by the use of a bronchodilator such as Bronkosol (isoetharine hydrochloride) or Ventolin (albuterol). Other side effects reported include a burning in the back of the throat, an unpleasant taste, brief lung spasms, and mild hypoglycemia.

Cautions Regarding the Usage of Pentamidine

There have been several recent reports about both new and secondary cases of PCP occurring in people being treated with aerosol pentamidine. As this book is being edited (June 1990), some physicians are beginning to believe that treatment with oral antibiotics such as Septra (trimethoprim-sulfamethoxazole) and Dapsone (diamino-diphenyl sulfone) is superior. However, these are much more toxic, so check with your physician before doing anything.

RIBAVIRIN

Ribavirin is a wide-spectrum antiviral drug that is sold in many countries. It is used to combat a variety of conditions, including herpes, flu, colds, and viral illness common in tropical regions.

Ribavirin is of the category of drugs called nucleoside analogues, as are AZT and acyclovir. These drugs work by creating a decoy substance which the virus mistakes for a protein that it uses in its reproductive cycle. When the virus links up with the decoy, the chain of reproduction is broken, since the decoy doesn't really contain what the virus needs to complete its reproduction.

In 1987 ribavirin became the subject of controversy between its manufacturer, ICN Pharmaceuticals, and the FDA. The FDA claimed that there was actually a disproportionate number of deaths among patients who took ribavirin in a study of patients with ARC, indicating that ribavirin had actually worsened the HIV infection. Although this was later disproved, the studies remain very controversial

More recent studies on the effects of ribavirin show a reduction of viral activity, improved immune response, and increased patient survival. It has been suggested that the drug is a less toxic alternative to the use of AZT.

Word-of-mouth reports on the use of ribavirin are generally positive, with the best results reported when the drug is used at the early stages of the disease. Most people considered it helpful in slowing the progress and symptoms of the HIV infection.

Recommended Dosage

Recommended dosages for ribavirin vary widely. As with any drug, some people are more sensitive to it than others, and may experience more and stronger side effects. The typical dosage is from four to twelve 200 milligram tablets per day. Only a few people can tolerate the highest dosages, while most can tolerate the lowest dose.

Side Effects of Ribavirin

Ribavirin has only minimal side effects compared to other nucleoside analogue types of antivirals. The most common side effect is anemia, which is related to the strength of the dosage taken. When anemia occurs, it is treated by dose reduction, and in all cases has been reversible.

Other common side effects include minor central nervous system disturbances, headaches, twitches, jitters, and insomnia. These are reportedly worsened by alcohol consumption.

CHAPTER XI

Conclusion

The FDA's policy change allowing mail-order importation of drugs marks the beginning of a revolution in how Americans obtain their health care treatments. I think that we, as a people, have now passed the peak of unnecessary control that we will have to endure from the government, medical, and pharmaceutical industry.

We owe most of our thanks for these changes to the activists in the gay rights movement working on the AIDS problem; the women's rights movement, concerned about pro choice; and the gray movement, who are concerned about the high costs of medical care along with the need for new treatments in the areas of senility, cancer, and overall aging.

Because of them we are started on a path that will lead to major changes in our pharmaceutical system. Over the next several years mail-order importation of foreign drugs will become common. More of our current prescription drugs will be made available over-the-counter. And the FDA will become more liberal in its approach to the drug approval process, as well as in its approach to what it attempts to ban from import.

We are bound to continue on this path for several reasons. First, the medical-pharmaceutical industry is going to come under even greater pressure from the special interest groups for AIDS, gray rights, and women's rights. These and other groups are going to demand that the FDA do things that are positive and that it speed up its overall drug approval process.

Second, the number of applications for approved drug status is going to increase greatly. These applications will involve more complicated drugs and more complicated issues. Finally, in an age defined by conservatism, it isn't likely that the FDA will get much additional funding. The FDA will be called on to do more things with relatively fewer resources.

Given all this, the FDA will either loosen up in its efforts to control things and its need to obsess over each drug it tests, or it will break down. In the end, after much hand wringing and doomsday talk, it will loosen up.

Signs of this loosening of control become evident almost every day that goes by. Today it is announced that the FDA is giving its official sanction to a controversial underground clinical study of Compound Q that was begun without proper approval. Tomorrow, the FDA will remove its import ban on RU 486 so that women can obtain safer abortions without the costs and risks associated with surgery.

The world is changing, and the FDA will have to change too. The people are demanding it. We all will be better off when this group has less time on its hands.

I am aware that many people will not totally agree with this position. Their views are understandable to me. There will always be at least a small question about whether it is better to have a cautious policy that limits the possibility of negative side effects from drugs not yet fully tested—or whether it is better to help the people who are sick today and worry about side effects tomorrow.

Ultimately, I suppose, the issue will come down to the seriousness of the diseases involved and the possible side effects of the treatments in question. But I am sure that sensible approval procedures can be developed that take both of these issues into account.

It is my hope that the facts presented in this book will get people started thinking about these concerns, and that this book will help them move toward a more independent approach to their own health care. But I also hope that this material helps us ordinary people finish the process that the activist groups got started, so that we end up with a medical-pharmaceutical system that truly does serve the needs of the population.

APPENDIX I

Guide to International Pharmaceutical Suppliers Including Sample Price Lists

Alan Pharmaceuticals, Ltd.
204 Essex Road
London N1 3AP England
Telephone: 44-01-226-
6246

Associated Pharmaceuti-
cals, Inc.
9 Atis Road
Malabon, Metro Manila,
Philippines
Telephone: 63-2-361-2649

John Bell & Croyden
54 Wigmore Street
London, WIH OAU
England
Telephone: 44-01-935-5555

Laboratories Bial Portela &
Ca. Lda.
Sede/Rua Joao Oliveira
Ramos, 87
4000 Porto-Portugal
Apartado 4037
Telephone: 351-493-054

Blue Ridge Pharmaceuticals
17 Natib
Mandaluyong, Metro
Manila, Philippines
Telephone: 63-2-773-372

Danmarks Apotekerforen-
ing
Bredgade 54
P.O. Box 2181
DK-1017 Copenhagen K.,
Denmark

Doctors Pharmaceuticals,
Inc.
345-B San Diego
Caloocan City, Metro
Manila, Philippines
Telephone: 63-2-345-971

Drugmaker's Laboratories,
Inc.
335 Sto. Rosario
Mangaluyong, Metro
Manila, Philippines
Telephone: 63-2-780-071

Elin Pharmaceuticals
115 Scout Rallos
Quezon City, Metro
   Manila Philippines
Telephone: 63-2-975-367

Evans Medical, Ltd.
Langhurst
Horsham, West Sussex
   RH12 4QD England
Telephone: 44-04-034-
   1400

A/S Ferrosan
5 Sydmarken
DK-2860 Soeborg,
   Denmark

Foreningen ad Danske
   Medicinfabrikker
Landemaerket 25
DK-1119 Copenhagen K.,
   Denmark .

Germed-export-import
Schicklerstrasse 5/7
Berlin DDR-1020
Telephone: 49-30-21-480

Lab Bial Portela & Ca.,
   Lda.
Sede/Rua Oliveira Ramos
   87
4000 Porto-Portugal,
   Apartado 4037
Telephone: 351-493-054

Maripharm, Ltd.
21, Varvaki Str.
114 74 Athens, Greece
Telephone: 30-01-641-
   1208

Mecobenzon A/S
29, Halmtorvet
DK-1503 Copenhagen,
   Denmark

Myra Pharm, Inc.
United
Mandaluyong, Metro
   Manila, Philippines
Telephone: 63-721-6501

Pharmaceuticals Interna-
   tional
539 Telegraph Canyon
   Rd., Suite 227
Chula Vista, California
   92010-6436
Telephone: 1-800-365-
   3698

Quimica Y Farmacia
66200 Monterrey N.L.
   Mexico

Reckitt & Colman
   (Overseas), Ltd.
Dansom Lane
Hull HU 8 7DS England
Telephone: 44-04-822-
   6151

Regent Laboratories, Ltd.
Letap House
861 Coronation Road
London NW10 7PT
   England
Telephone: 44-01-961-
   6868

The Wallis Laboratory,
   Ltd.
11 Camford Way
Sundon Park
Luton LU3 3AN England
Telephone: 44-050-258-
   4884

The following suppliers furnished price lists that can be
used for reference purposes.

B. Mougios & Co. O.E.
Pittakou 23 T.K.
54645
Thessaloniki, Greece
Telephone: 30-03-185-
   9680

Bomuca SA De CV
Avenue De Los Pollos
   26-C
La Mesa, Tijuana, B.C.,
   Mexico 22456
Telephone: 52-66-216074
Fax: 52-66-216075

Masters Marketing Co.,
   Ltd.
Masters House
No. 1 Marlborough Hill
Harrow, Middlesex HA1
   1TW England
Telephone: 44-01-427-
   9978
Telex: 940-11062-MAST
   G
Fax: 44-01-427-1994

Vipharm Pharmaceutical
  Products E. Tsati & Co.
35, Agorakritou Street
104 40 Athens, Greece
Telephone: 30-01-883-
  1680 and 30-01-822-
  7685
Telex: 222278 ELPA GR.
Fax: 30-01-883-1680

John Bell & Croyden
54 Wigmore St.
London, England W1H
  OAU
Telephone: 44-01-935-
  5555
Telex: 89-55447-JBell-G

SAMPLE PRICE LISTS

Following are some examples of what you can expect as far as ordering practices and prices of companies abroad. We publish these lists as they were received from the companies, as of January 1, 1990, and are not responsible for price changes or policies that may have occurred since this publication.

Note: The drugs in this section are listed by brand name, with generic name(s) in parentheses. For a detailed description of these medications, refer to the alphabetically listed generic names in chapters VII, VIII, IX, and X.

B. Mougios & Co. O.E.
Pittakou 23 T.K.
54645
Thessaloniki, Greece
Telephone: 30-03-185-9680

Ordering instructions: Payment should be by cashier's check or money order. Call to see if they accept credit cards. Include $5 additional for shipping and handling. Delivery will be within four weeks.

Zovirax (acyclovir)
    25 tablets, 200 milligrams $75.00
    cream, 2 grams 5 percent   16.00
    cream, 10 grams 5 percent   48.00

Amoxil or Paradroxil (amoxicillin)
    12 capsules, 500 milligrams   3.00
    100 capsules, 500 milligrams   34.00
    80 tablets, 1 gram disp.   52.00
    suspension, 60 milliliters 250 milligrams
        per 5 milliliters   6.00
    suspension, 60 milliliters 500 milligrams
        per 5 milliliters   7.50
    vial, 250 milligram solution   3.50
    vial, 500 milligram solution   4.50
    vial, 1 gram solution   5.50

Pentrexyl (ampicillin)
    12 capsules, 500 milligrams   3.00
    100 capsules, 500 milligrams   28.00
    100 tablets, 1 gram   45.00

Augmentin (amoxicillin plus clavulanic acid)
    12 tablets SISP 625 milligrams   21.00
    syrup, 60 milliliters 156, 25 milligrams
        per 5 milliliters   12.00

Septra (sulfamethoxazole-trimethoprim)
    10 tablets, 960 milligrams   6.00
    syrup, 100 milliliters pediatric
        (5 per 240 milligrams)   9.00
    syrup, 100 milliliters forte
        (5 per 480 milligrams)   16.00

Ceclor (cefaclor)
    12 capsules, 500 milligrams $23.00
    suspension, 60 milliliters 125 milligrams
        per 5 milliliters   13.00
    suspension, 60 milliliters 250 milligrams
        per 5 milliliters   19.00

Adalat or Glopir (nifedipine)
    50 capsules, 5 milligrams   13.00
    50 capsules, 10 milligrams   18.00
    30 capsules, 20 milligrams time-release   15.00

Duvadilan (isoxsuprine hydrochloride)
    50 tablets, 20 milligrams   7.00
    60 capsules, 40 milligrams time-release   15.00

Loniten (minoxidil)
    100 tablets, 5 milligrams   31.00
    100 tablets, 10 milligrams   60.00

Nitrong (nitroglycerin)
    30 tablets, 2.6 milligrams   10.00
    30 tablets, 6.5 milligrams   17.00

Tagamet (cimetidine)
    50 tablets, 200 milligrams   17.00
    25 tablets, 400 milligrams   18.00
    15 tablets, 800 milligrams   17.00
    2 milliliters, 200 milligrams   12.00

Zantac (ranitidine hydrochloride)
    20 tablets, 150 milligrams   20.00
    10 tablets, 300 milligrams   17.00

Zyloric (allopurinol)
    25 tablets, 100 milligrams   3.50
    28 tablets, 300 milligrams   7.50

Tenormin (atenolol)
28 tablets, 50 milligrams
(50 per 12.5) milligrams $9.00
8 tablets, 100 milligrams
(50 per 25) milligrams   12.00

Loftyl (buflomedil hydrochloride)
30 tablets, 150 milligrams   9.50
20 tablets, 300 milligrams   12.00
drops, 20 milliliters 150 milligrams
per milliliter   11.00
suspension, 50 milligrams IV   7.00

Capoten (captopril)
20 tablets, 25 milligrams   8.50
20 tablets, 50 milligrams   17.00
20 tablets, 100 milligrams   30.00

Catapres (clonidine hydrochloride)
30 tablets, 15 milligrams   3.00
suspension, 15 milligrams per milliliter   6.00

Pancoran transdermal (nitroglycerin)
30 pieces, 25 milligrams per 10 centimeters   24.00
30 pieces, 50 milligrams per 20 centimeters   45.00

Pensordil (isosorbide dinitrate)
30 capsules, 20 milligrams time-release   6.00
30 capsules, 40 milligrams time-release   7.00
50 tablets, 3.5 milligrams sublingual   5.00
40 tablets, 5 milligrams sublingual   5.00

Ceporex or Keflex (cephalexin)
12 capsules, 500 milligrams   9.00
suspension, 60 milliliters 250 milligrams
per 5 milliliters   10.00
suspension, 60 milliliters 500 milligrams
per 5 milliliters   10.00

Flagyl (metronidazole hydrochloride)
   30 capsules, 500 milligrams $10.00
   suspension, 120 milliliters 4 percent   10.00
   10 vaginal tablets, 500 milligrams   7.00
   10 ovules, 500 milligrams   7.50

Lincocin (lincomycin hydrochloride monohydrate)
   12 capsules, 500 milligrams   11.00
   syrup, 60 milliliters 250 milligrams
     per 5 milliliters   11.00
   vial, 600 milligrams 2 milliliters   5.00

Daktarin (miconazole nitrate)
   20 tablets, 250 milligrams   12.00
   oral gel   7.00
   cream, 30 grams 2 percent   7.00
   tincture, 30 milliliters   7.00
   lotion, 30 milliliters   7.00
   powder, 20 grams 2 percent   6.00
   vaginal cream, 78 grams 2 percent,
    16 applications   15.00
   ovules, 200 grams   15.00
   ovules, 400 grams   14.00

Phenergan (promethazine hydrochloride)
   20 tablets, 25 milligrams   2.00
   syrup, 125 milliliters   5.50
   cream, 30 grams 2 percent   3.00
   syrup, 2 grams 50 milligrams   5.00

Glucophage (metformin hydrochloride)
   30 tablets, 750 milligrams time-release   5.00

Diamox (acetazolamide)
   100 tablets, 250 milligrams   11.00

Lasix (frusemide)
    30 capsules, 30 milligrams time-release $6.00
    12 capsules, 40 milligrams   5.00
    syrup, 2 milliliters 10 milligrams per milliliter 6.00

Dulcolax (bisacodyl)
    30 tablets, 5 milligrams   2.00
    6 suppositories adult, 10 milligrams   2.00

Imodium (loperamide hydrochloride)
    6 capsules, 2 milligrams   2.50
    drops, 10 milliliters 2 milligrams per milliliter 3.50

Polysilane (dimethicone)
    30 sachets, 15 grams   8.00

Laxatol (sodium picosulfate)
    24 capsules, 7.5 milligrams   3.00
    24 toffees, 5 milligrams   3.00
    drops, 10 milliliters   2.50

Gastrozepin (pirenzepine hydrochloride)
    30 tablets, 25 milligrams   8.00
    5 ampoules, 10 milligrams   14.00

Nonzinan (levomepromazine)
    20 tablets, 25 milligrams   4.00

Cilroton (domperidone)
    30 tablets, 10 milligrams   7.50
    solution, 200 milliliters 1 milligram
       per milliliter   11.00
    drops, 30 milliliters 10 milligrams per milliliter 9.00
    6 suppositories, 10 milligrams   4.00
    6 suppositories, 30 milligrams   5.00
    6 suppositories, 60 milligrams   8.00

Zaditen (ketotifen fumarate)
   30 tablets, 1 gram $12.00
   syrup, 60 milliliters   13.00

Terramycin (oxytetracycline)
   100 capsules, 250 milligrams   17.00
   10 vaginal tablets, 100 milligrams   4.00

Ospen (penicillin V potassium)
   40 tablets, 1,500,000 IU   16.00
   60 milliliter suspension, 400,000 IU
      per 5 milliliters   8.00
   60 milliliter suspension, 750,000 IU
      per 5 milliliters   9.50

Vidarabine (vidarabine phosphate)
   ointment, 10 grams 3 percent   27.00
   eye ointment, 5 grams 3 percent   18.00

Tofranil (imipramine hydrochloride)
   60 tablets, 10 milligrams   3.00
   50 tablets, 25 milligrams   3.50

Delta-Cortef or Prezolon (prednisolone)
   100 tablets, 5 milligrams   12.00
   30 tablets, 5 milligrams   4.00
   3 ampoules, 25 milligrams   10.00

Thyrostat (carbimazole)
   100 tablets, 5 milligrams   5.00

Nebacetin (neomycin sulfate with bacitracin)
   ointment, 15 grams   5.50
   powder, 5 grams   4.50
   powder spray, 200 grams   20.00
   powder sterile, 50 grams   13.00
   eye ointment, 2.5 grams   4.00
   collodion, 10 milliliters   7.00

Furadantin or Macrodantin (nitrofurantoin)

25 tablets, 50 milligrams	$5.00
12 tablets, 100 milligrams	5.00
30 capsules, 50 milligrams	6.00
30 capsules, 100 milligrams	8.00

Mycostatin (nystatin)

12 tablets, 500,000 IU	3.00
suspension, 12 doses	3.50
cream, 15 grams	5.00
ointment, 15 grams, 100,000 IU	5.00
powder, 20 grams	3.50
15 vaginal tablets	3.50
vaginal cream, 32 grams	6.00

Bomuca SA De CV
Avenue De Los Pollos 26-C
La Mesa, Tijuana, B.C., Mexico 22456
Telephone: 52-66-216074
Fax: 52-66-216075

Ordering instructions: Use your credit card or send a personal check or money order. Add $6.50 for shipping and handling. Ask about next day delivery. Call for information about medications not on this list.

Diflucan (fluconazole)

1 capsule, 150 milligrams	$30.74
7 capsules, 50 milligrams	71.56

Lomidine (pentamadine)

5 vials, 300 milligrams	225.00

Tribavirin (ribavirin)

12 tablets, 200 milligrams	19.50

Masters Marketing Co., Ltd.
Masters House
No. 1 Marlborough Hill
Harrow, Middlesex HA1 1TW England
Telephone: 44-01-427-9978
Telex: 940-11062-MAST G
Fax: 44-01-427-1994

Ordering instructions: An order of $100 US will include the shipping cost by air parcel post. For amounts of less than $100, an extra charge of $10 will be made for shipping. Payment by a US draft (cashier's check or money order) should be included with the order. Goods are of UK and European origin. The brand names as shown will be supplied.

Zovirax (acyclovir)
cream, 2 grams 5 percent	$18.31
cream, 10 grams 5 percent	55.21
ointment, 4.5 grams 3 percent	23.35
suspension, 125 milliliters	72.71
25 tablets, 200 milligrams	72.71
56 tablets, 400 milligrams	266.71

Amoxycillin
100 capsules, 200 milligrams	29.94
100 capsules, 500 milligrams	57.64
pediatric syrup, 100 milliliters per 125 milligrams	47.73
adult syrup, 500 milliliters per 250 milligrams	87.60

Ampicillin
500 capsules, 250 milligrams	35.22
250 capsules, 500 milligrams	35.22
pediatric syrup, 100 milliliters per 125 milligrams	15.36
adult syrup, 100 milliliters per 250 milligrams	22.70

Augmentin (amoxicillin trihydrate + clavulanic acid)
  100 tablets, 375 milligrams $80.93
   21 tablets, 375 milligrams   16.79
  junior suspension, 100 milliliters   9.89
  pediatric suspension, 100 milliliters   7.85

Distaclor (cefaclor)
  100 capsules, 250 milligrams   109.26

Ceporex (cephalexin)
  100 capsules, 250 milligrams   38.44
  100 capsules, 500 milligrams   75.24

Orbenin (cloxacillin)
  100 capsules, 250 milligrams   45.26
  100 capsules, 500 milligrams   91.73
  syrup, 100 milliliters per 125 milligrams   7.95

Flucloxacillin
  100 capsules, 250 milligrams   27.48
  100 capsules, 500 milligrams   59.21
  syrup, 100 milliliters per 125 milligrams   76.13

Hiprex (hexamine hippurate)
  60 tablets, 1 gram   11.68

Flagyl (metronidazole hydrochloride)
  21 tablets, 200 milligrams   5.16
  14 tablets, 400 milligrams   7.32

Lincocin (lincomycin hydrochloride monohydrate)
   12 capsules, 500 milligrams   18.52
  100 capsules, 500 milligrams   145.39
  syrup, 200 milligrams per 5 milliliters   19.00

257

Daktarin (miconazole nitrate)
cream, 15 grams 2 percent $3.19
oral gel, 40 grams 6.28
oral tablets, 20 grams 37.48
powder, 20 grams 2 percent 3.19
spray powder, 100 grams 3.19

Furadantin (nitrofurantoin)
suspension, 300 milliliters 11.31
100 tablets, 50 milligrams 22.07
100 tablets, 500 milligrams 42.45

Mycostatin (nystatin)
suspension, 30 milliliters 6.28
cream, 15 grams 3.90
gel, 30 grams 6.69
ointment, 15 grams 2.74
28 tablets 6.21
28 pastilles 9.94
100 pessaries 17.61

Terramycin (oxytetracycline)
28 capsules, 250 milligrams 2.41

Stabillin VK (penicillin V potassium)
elixir, 62.5 milligrams per 5 milliliters 1.01
elixir, 125 milligrams per 5 milliliters 1.26
elixir, 250 milligrams per 5 milliliters 2.01

Vira-A (vidarabine phosphate opthalmin)
ointment, 3.5 grams 16.05

Tofranil (imipramine hydrochloride)
500 tablets, 10 milligrams 8.55
1000 tablets, 25 milligrams 13.87

Precortisyl (prednisolone)
    500 tablets, 1 milligram $5.62
    1000 tablets, 5 milligrams   17.37
    500 tablets, 2.5 milligrams   11.00

Decortisyl (prednisone)
    500 tablets, 1 milligram   5.13
    1000 tablets, 5 milligrams   17.40

Neomercazole (carbimazole)
    100 tablets, 20 milligrams   22.47
    100 tablets, 5 milligrams   6.07

Piriton (chlorpheniramine)
    500 tablets, 4 milligrams   11.60
    30 tablets, 4 milligrams   1.57
    syrup, 150 milliliters   .72

Phenergan (promethazine hydrochloride)
    56 tablets, 10 milligrams   2.40
    25 tablets, 25 milligrams   3.57
    elixir, 100 milliliters   2.62

Orabet (metformin hydrochloride)
    100 tablets, 500 milligrams   4.75
    60 tablets, 850 milligrams   4.62

Diamox (acetazolamide)
    100 tablets, 25 milligrams   26.37

Aprinox (bendrofluazide)
    500 tablets, 2.5 milligrams   6.95
    1000 tablets, 5.5 milligrams   6.00

Lasix (frusemide)
    28 tablets, 20 milligrams   2.10
    28 tablets, 40 milligrams   3.65
    100 tablets, 500 milligrams   146.70

Dulcolax (bisacodyl)
  60 tablets, 5 milligrams $4.32
  20 suppositories, 10 milligrams   4.88

Imodium (loperamide hydrochloride)
  12 capsules, 2 milligrams   3.78
  30 capsules, 2 milligrams   8.40
  syrup, 100 milliliters   4.75

Gastrozepin (pirenzepine hydrochloride)
  60 tablets, 50 milligrams   51.25

Picolax (sodium picosulfate)
  sachets, 25 treatments   37.13

Tagamet (cimetidine)
  syrup, 600 milliliters   64.75
  50 tablets, 200 milligrams   21.42
  20 tablets, 400 milligrams   17.90
  60 tablets, 400 milligrams   46.72
  80 tablets, 800 milligrams   44.40

Zantac (ranitidine hydrochloride)
  syrup, 300 milliliters 150 milligrams
    per 10 milliliters   55.50
  60 tablets, 150 milligrams   74.40
  30 tablets, 300 milligrams   68.57

Zyloric (allopurinol)
  100 tablets, 100 milligrams   50.75
  30 tablets, 300 milligrams   39.00

Atropine Sulfate
  100 tablets, 600 milligrams   14.12

Capoten (captopril)
  100 tablets, 12.5 milligrams $47.15
  56 tablets, 25 milligrams   30.07
  56 tablets, 50 milligrams   51.25

Dixarit (clonidine hydrochloride)
  112 tablets, 25 milligrams   15.32

Adalate (nifedepine)
  90 capsules, 10 milligrams   27.42
  50 tablets, 20 milligrams time-release   24.13

Loniten (minoxidil)
  100 tablets, 2.5 milligrams   29.50
  100 tablets, 5 milligrams   53.15
  100 tablets, 10 milligrams   102.95

Nitroglycerin
  100 capsules, 500 milligrams   21.60

Sorbide Nitrate (isosorbide dinitrate)
  100 tablets, 10 milligrams   2.98

Persantine (dipyridamole)
  100 tablets, 25 milligrams   7.87
  100 tablets, 100 milligrams   20.87

Inderal (propranolol hydrochloride)
  100 tablets, 10 milligrams   2.50
  100 tablets, 40 milligrams   6.75
  100 tablets, 80 milligrams   6.60
  100 tablets, 160 milligrams   11.70

Serpasil (reserpine)
  100 tablets, 1 milligram   1.18
  100 tablets, .25 milligram   2.42

Eumovate (clobetasone butyrate)
cream/ointment, 30 grams $4.40
eye drops, 10 milliliters 7.60
eye drops with neomycin, 10 milliliters 6.75

Hexopal (inositol nicotinate)
100 tablets, 500 milligrams 48.92
112 tablets, 750 milligrams 81.15
suspension, 300 milliliters 1 gram
per 5 milliliters 49.75

Eradicin (acrosoxacin)
20 capsules, 150 milligrams 72.60

Treosulfan
100 capsules, 250 milligrams 75.28

Mismanal (astemizole)
30 tablets, 10 milligrams 13.12

Motilium (domperidone)
30 tablets, 10 milligrams 6.12

Comprecin (enoxacin)
6 tablets, 200 milligrams 13.50

Zaditen (ketotifen)
60 tablets, 1 milligram 29.83
elixir, 150 milliliters 17.63

Clarityn (loratidine)
30 tablets, 10 milligrams 27.00

Cytotec (misoprostol)
56 tablets, 200 micrograms 32.50

Tenormin (atenolol)
28 tablets, 50 milligrams $10.47
28 tablets, 100 milligrams 15.10

Cordilox (verapamil hydrochloride)
56 tablets, 120 milligrams 19.67
100 tablets, 40 milligrams 11.72
100 tablets, 80 milligrams 23.45
28 tablets, 160 milligrams 26.22
28 tablets, 240 milligrams 27.30

Marevan (warfarin)
100 tablets, 1 milligram 1.45
100 tablets, 3 milligrams 1.80
100 tablets, 5 milligrams 2.85

Voltaren (diclofenac)
30 tablets, 25 milligrams 7.04
30 tablets, 50 milligrams 13.68
30 100 milligrams time-release 16.73

Canestan (clotrimazole)
cream, 10 grams 1 percent 4.55
vaginal cream, 35 grams 2 percent 13.05
6 vaginal tablets, 100 milligrams 6.60
3 vaginal tablets, 200 milligrams 6.45
solution, 20 milliliters 5.95
powder, 30 grams 3.90

Synalar (fluocinolone acetonide)
cream, 15 grams 1.95
gel, 15 grams 3.75
ointment, 15 grams 1.95

Synalar C (fluocinolone acetonide with clioquinol)
cream, 15 grams 2.40
ointment, 15 grams 2.40

Synalar N (fluocinolone acetonide with neomycin)
  cream, 15 grams $2.08
  ointment, 15 grams   2.08

Retin-A (retinoic acid)
  cream, 60 grams .01 percent   14.13
  cream, 60 grams .25 percent   14.13
  cream, 60 grams .05 percent   14.13

Hydrocortisone
  cream/ointment, 15 grams .5 percent   .88
  cream/ointment, 15 grams 1.0 percent   1.05
  cream/ointment, 30 grams 1.0 percent   1.88

Retrovir (AZT)
  100 capsules, 100 milligrams   229.20
  40 capsules, 250 milligrams   229.20

Septra (trimethoprim-sulfamethoxazole)
  100 tablets, 480 milligrams   41.72
  suspension, adult 100 milliliters   11.85
  suspension, pediatric, 100 milliliters   6.55

Acetyldigitoxin
  500 tablets, 60.5 micrograms   4.87
  1000 tablets, 25 micrograms   6.65
  1000 tablets, 250 micrograms   10.27

Vipharm Pharmaceutical Products, E. Tsati & Co.
35, Agorakritou Street
104 40 Athens, Greece
Telephone: 30-01-88-31-680 or 30-01-822-7685
Telex: 222278 ELPA GR.
Fax: 30-01-883-1680

Associated with
Olympia Skouvaras, Pharmacy
Epaminonda 82, Thivai, Greece
Telephone: 30-01-822-7685
Fax: 30-01-883-1680

Shown here are wholesale prices. To the best of our knowledge, this pharmacy is willing to fill personal orders as well. You may have to write, fax, or call to confirm prices on personal (three-month) quantities of any given drug.

Ordering instructions: Their instructions are: "Transfer money at sight by swift or telex." They will accept a money order made out to Vipharm & Co. Or you may go to your bank and transfer the payment directly to their account. Their bank is the Commercial Bank of Greece, Branch N. 012, 100 Acharnon Street, Athens 10434 Greece, Telex: 218787.

Zovirax (acyclovir)
  25 tablets, 200 milligrams
    10 cases 250 tablets $835.00
  5 vials, 250 milligrams
    5 cases 25 vials   825.00
  2 grams 5 percent cream
    15 cases 15 tubes   253.00
  10 grams 5 percent cream
    15 cases 15 tubes   750.00

Augmentin (amoxicillin plus clavulanic acid)
  12 tablets, 625 milligrams
    20 cases 240 tablets   413.00

Pentrexl (ampicillin)
  100 capsules, 500 milligrams
    10 cases 1000 capsules   268.00
  100 capsules, 1 gram
    10 cases 1000 capsules   428.00

Tofranil (imipramine hydrochloride)
  50 tablets, 25 milligrams
    20 cases 1000 tablets $513.00

Glopir (nifedipine)
  50 tablets, 10 milligrams
    30 cases 1000 tablets   164.00
  30 tablets, 20 milligrams
    20 cases 600 tablets   238.00

Loniten (minoxidil)
  100 tablets, 5 milligrams
    20 cases 2000 tablets   574.00
  100 tablets, 10 milligrams
    20 cases 2000 tablets   1,040.00

Rogaine Solution (for hair restoral)
  60 milliliters 2 percent
    5 cases 5 bottles   335.00

Pancoran (nitroglycerin)
  30 patches, 25 milligrams per 10 centimeters
    5 cases 450 patches   397.00
  30 patches, 50 milligrams per 20 centimeters
    5 cases 450 patches   699.00

Ceclor (cefaclor)
  12 capsules, 500 milligrams
    20 cases 240 capsules   421.00

Lincocin (lincomycin hydrochloride monohydrate)
  12 capsules, 500 milligrams
    20 cases 240 capsules   199.00

Vidarabine
  ointment, 10 grams 3 percent
    20 cases 20 tubes $525.00
  eye ointment, 5 grams 3 percent
    20 cases 20 tubes   337.00

Tenormin (atenolol)
  21 tablets, 100 milligrams
    20 cases 2100 tablets   243.00

John Bell & Croyden
54 Wigmore Street
London W1H OAU England
Telephone: 44-01-935-5555
Telex: 89-55447-JBell-G

Bonjela Antiseptic Oral Gel—8.7 percent choline
  salicylate, 0.01 percent cetalkonium chloride
  10 gram tube $1.90

Transvasin Cream
  2.0 percent ethylnicotinate, 2.0 percent
    hexylnicotinate, 14.0 percent tetrahydrofurfuryl
    salicylate, 2.0 percent benzocaine
    30 gram tube   1.15

Lloyd's Cream
  (diethylamine salicylate 10 percent)
    30 gram tube   1.40
    100 gram jar   2.72

Timoped Cream
  (tolnaftate BP 1.0 percent, triclosan 0.25 percent)
    30 gram tube   8.82

Timocort Hydrocortisone Cream
  (hydrocortisone BP 1 percent)
    15 gram tube   2.40

APPENDIX II

Abridged Copies of All Recent FDA Import Alerts That Are Related to the Mail-Order Importation of Drugs

Alert No. 66-41
August 1, 1988
ALL UNAPPROVED NEW DRUGS PROMOTED IN THE US
REASON FOR ALERT:

Media reports concerning the referenced pilot guidance for release of mail importation have inaccurately suggested that any unapproved drug may be imported through the mail for personal use. The pilot guidance is much more restrictive than reported. The pilot guidance was intended to be applicable only to (1) persons who have received treatment in a foreign country and who, upon returning to the United States, have imported the drug for their personal use in an effort to continue the treatment started abroad; and (2) persons who have made their own arrangements for obtaining drugs from foreign sources when that drug has not been promoted in the United States.

Whenever there is evidence of promotion of unapproved drugs to persons in the United States, the products should be detained. Evidence of promotion may consist of solicitations for mail orders, press releases, advertising materials, and other public announcements that are directed to persons residing in the US.

Paragraph 5 of the pilot guidance was intended to recommend import alerts when the promotion of an unapproved product falls within CPS 7150.10 (the Compliance Policy Guide) on health fraud. Thus, the field may recommend import alerts when a product meets the criteria for either a direct health hazard or an indirect health hazard.

The gist of the message is that all current import alerts restricting fraudulent, dangerous, and commercial drug importations will continue to be in effect in spite of what anyone thinks about the new mail import policy. You cannot bring in anything that has previously been on import alert.

Alert No. 57-02 Revised
January 30, 1986
TUBERCULOSIS VACCINE or MARUYAMA VACCINE
REASON FOR ALERT:

During 1977, Chicago, New York, and Seattle (Anchorage Airport) detained an unlicensed biologic (tuberculosis vaccine) from Japan. The vaccine is also known as Maruyama vaccine. This product was found in the personal luggage of tourists returning to this country. A *National Enquirer* article reported this product as having been used with success in the cure of certain types of cancer in Japan by Dr. Maruyama.

Dr. Haruo Sugano, Director, Cancer Research Institute of Japan has advised that Dr. Maruyama's vaccine is still experimental and of questionable efficacy against cancer.

The scientific community in Japan has not

accepted Dr. Maruyama's vaccine; tests of the vaccine in animals indicated it is not effective against cancer.

GUIDANCE:

This drug can only be obtained through a physician who has a "Notice of Claimed Investigational Exemption for a New Drug" for Maruyama vaccine on file with the Office of Biologics Research and Review, National Center for Drugs and Biologics, Food and Drug Administration. Only one IND remained active as of the data of this alert, Dr. K. Kuo H. Taira.

When shipments of Maruyama vaccine are encountered that are not covered by the above IND sponsor, ascertain the name and address of the receiving physician and contact the Division of Biological Investigational New Drugs to determine if an IND has been filed since this alert was issued.

Alert No. 57-03 Revised
January 30, 1986
HERPES VIRUS VACCINE (LUPIDON G AND LUPIDON H)
REASON FOR ALERT:

The FDA in New York City obtained information in 1976 that unlicensed biologics (herpes virus vaccines) were entering the United States via personal baggage. The vaccines are known as Lupidon G (for herpes type 2 infection) and Lupidon H (for herpes type 1 infection), and are manufactured by Herbal0Chemic, Hamburg, Germany.

Another manufacturer/shipper, Comptoir Pharmaceutique, Luxembourg, has also shipped Lupidon G to the United States via personal mail.

Alert local customs officials that if these drugs

are found, they should be reported to FDA. These drugs can only be legally obtained through a physician who has a "Notice of Claimed Investigational Exemption for a New Drug" on file with the Office of Biologics Research and Review Center, Food and Drug Administration.

Currently, clinical studies have not been approved for either vaccine. Therefore, when shipments of these vaccines are encountered, ascertain the name and address of the receiving physician and contact the Division of Biological Investigation, New Drugs, to determine if an IND has been subsequently filed. All entries for Lupidon G and Lupidon H not covered by an IND should be detained, etc.

Alert No. 66-27 Revised
February 26, 1987
ALL DRUGS FROM THE HAUPTMANN
INSTITUTE, VIENNA, AUSTRIA

Centrophenoxiene, Clonidine, Conjunctasin A Eyedrops, Eludril (mouthwash), Encefalux 60, Ethoxyquin, Hydergine Ergoloid mesylates, Gerovital GH3, Gerovital GH3 injectable, Gerovital GH3 face cream, KH3, Isoprinosine, Levodopa Sinemet, Lucidril, Minoxidil 3 percent lotion (Biominx), Parlodel (Bromocriptine), Propranolol, Piracetam (Regenersen) RN-13, RN-13 (Neygeront), Retin-A cream, Syntopressin nasal spray, Tetracycline, Vasopressin, Zovirax cream

REASON FOR ALERT:

This alert covers drugs from the Hauptmann Institute, Vienna, Austria. The alert stated that Karl-Gustav Hauptmann, M.D., director of this firm, had purchased the Longevity Institute, S.A., Balboa, Republic of Panama. The "Institute" was founded to "liberate Americans and citizens of other countries from the tyranny of governments that choose to deny them the therapies essential to their health and longevity." While many of these drugs have domestic approval, the claims included in promotional labeling distributed by "The Institute" include conditions for which they are unapproved. . . .

Based on labeling, all of the above drugs are misbranded, because they lack adequate directions for use and include false and misleading claims. Such drugs are limited to prescription use and may be potentially lethal if improperly administered or if taken without adequate directions for use and without the supervision of a licensed practitioner.

Alert No. 66-28 Revised
December 10, 1987
UNAPPROVED NEW DRUGS PROMOTED BY DR. HANS NIEPER OF WEST GERMANY

Acetaldehyde, Anavit-F3, Argutin, Ascorbic Acid, Astenile, Benzalde E, Berigloobin, Bromelain, Calcium EAP, Calcipot-F and C, phosphate, Calciretard, Calcium-EAP, Calcium-ORO, Carnitin, Carnivora, Carnivora-VF, Carotaben, Cesium Chloride, Chol-Kugeletten, Coroverlan, Corticoide, Didrovaltrate, Dionacea Muscipula, Dona 200-S, E-mulsine Fertissimun, Enzynorm, Erogocalciferol, Eugalan Topfer, Fermento, Floracit-Gummetten, Fluoro-Uracil, Fucus Vesiculosis, Gallen-Leber-Tee-N, Glandul-Supra-Renal, Harnosal, Helixor, Hepaticum-Medice, Hornosal, Intralipid, Inzelloval, Iskodor, Ixoten, Kalinor-Brausetabletten, Kupferorotat, Lebertrankapseln, Lexotanil 6, Lithiumorotat, Lyndiol, Magagrisevit, Magnesium-Mangil, Magnesium Orotat

(Magnerot) Magnesium Verla, Mendelonitril Nicot, Mandelonitril ureat, Methotrexate, Millevit, Noradral Retard, Omniflora, Panzynorm, Pepsaletten, Pernical Forte, Pexan Forte, Phosetamin, Phosphatamin, Plv, Mandelonitrille, Prednoson-Ratiopharm, Predni-Tablinen, Progresin Retard, Purinetten forte, Resisticell, Selenium Chrol-Sride-H, Sol. Calciferol, Solu-Decortin-H, Sorbit, Spasmo-Harnosal, Squalen Purum, Standinol with Calcium, EAP and Phosetamin, Sterofundin, Sulf. Redox, Talusin, Taurin, Theo-Talusin, Thym-Uvocal, Thymus Extract, Thymus Multi, Thymus Uvocal, Tombusan, Traumanase forte, Trophicard-Kohler, Ungt. Rad. Valerianae, Valmane, Vegantobetten, Venostasin, Warnhlnwols Dieses, Arzneimittel, Wobenzym, Wobe-Mugos, Zink-Aspartat, Zinkorotat, Zyloric

REASON FOR ALERT:

Dr. Hans A. Nieper is an internist practicing "eumetabolic therapy" operating from the Paracelsus Silbersee Hospital, Hannover-Langenhagen, Federal Republic of Germany. He claims to have treated thousands of Americans—those who cannot be helped by orthodox medicine—for conditions including cancer, heart disease, and multiple sclerosis. Almost always, drugs promoted by Hans Nieper are labeled in German with no English language labeling and seldom do they contain directions for use.

Dr. Nieper attracts patients by using promotional material and by making speaking visits to the US. The agency's enforcement strategy regarding the handling of unapproved new drugs promoted by Dr. Nieper has included advising Dr. Nieper, the West German shippers of these drugs, and domestic promoters of Nieper's treatment regimen of the illegal status of these drugs in the US; contacting the US embassy in Bonn, Germany, and the West German government to determine what assistance they can provide in stopping the shipments of those products at their source; developing public information and educational materials in conjunction with major national and international health organizations; and requesting the US Customs Service and other government agencies to include information about foreign fraudulent health schemes and the importation of misbranded and unapproved new drugs and devices in their traveler's information pamphlets.

The majority of the initiatives in the enforcement strategy have now been completed. We have received a response from Dr. Nieper in which he stated that he believes that World Health Organization regulations or international law permit the importation of drugs that have been prescribed in another country if treatment was begun in that country. This, however, has been refuted by the World Health Organization.

Alert No. 66-03 Revised
March 25, 1986
CELLULAR THERAPY (NIEHANS CELL THERAPY; SICCACELL THERAPY)
REASON FOR ALERT:
Cellular therapy was developed by a Swiss physician, Paul Niehans, over twenty years ago. The products are primarily dried fetal animal tissues obtained from the heart, thymus, placenta, ovary, brain, and thyroid gland. They are intended for injection in the treatment of a multitude of human disease conditions. Siccacell-brand preparations were initially produced by

Pharmakon Ltd., Zurich, Switzerland. Cell therapy preparations have subsequently been manufactured by other European firms such as Bio-Pharm, West Germany.

In the late 1950s, these preparations were imported for investigational use in this country. However, data establishing the safety and efficacy for their recommended uses was never received by this Agency (FDA). A February 13, 1960 article published in the *Journal of the American Medical Association* raised serious questions concerning such preparations. The article implied that the medical theory was unsound and that such products were capable of causing harm.

We regard such preparations to be "new drugs" as defined in 21 USC 321 (p). There is no approved new drug application or acceptable IND permitting their use in this country at this time. Therefore, distribution in interstate commerce is not permitted.

We have seen a recent resurgence of marketing of such products in this country especially for use by "nutritional therapists" and "holistic practitioners." Mail entries from Europe appear to be the most common route into domestic commerce. Such shipments are commonly labeled in the German language and are destined to individuals. US Customs advises that frequent mail entries of cellular therapies are being received from the following West German shippers: 1. Franz Schmid, Ziegleberg, West Germany; 2. Varinwinkler, Heidelberg, West Germany; and 3. * H(M)aenina, Neckarsheinach, West Germany. Detain all such products offered for entry in the form of fetal tissue powders or extracts intended for injection.

Alert No. 56-01
February 19, 1982
CHLORAMPHENICOL WITHOUT NADA
REASON FOR ALERT:

Chloramphenicol, a certifiable antibiotic, needs an effective New Animal Drug Application (NADA) to be imported into this country. The product is cleared for use in the treatment of nonfood producing animals (dogs and cats).

There are no foreign manufacturers of chloramphenicol that have an effective NADA (Zenith Laboratories, St. Croix, Virgin Islands, does have an approved NADA for chloramphenicol capsules).

We have recently received reports that 500 milligrams per milliliter chloramphenicol solution is being imported into the US hidden in horse carriers. This concentration exceeds any level approved domestically and is probably intended in the labeling for use in food-producing animals and horses.

Detain all entries (formal or informal) of animal chloramphenicol manufactured by foreign firms (except Zenith Laboratories, St. Croix, Virgin Islands).

Alert No. 61-01
September 17, 1982
**GEROVITAL (KH3, CH3 etc), PROCAINE
  HYDROCHLORIDE**
REASON FOR ALERT:

KH2 and similar products marketed under various other names such as CH3, Procaine HCl, Gerovital, Trofibial H3, Asiavital, have been the subject of import alerts numbered 61-01, 61-02, and 61-03. This import alert updates and combines these three alerts into one.

KH3 generally consists of some form of Procaine HCL (injectable, tablets, powder, etc.). Procaine HCL is regarded as a new drug for all indications when offered for the conditions for which it was found effective under DESI 763. It requires an approved Abbreviated New Drug Application (ANDA) for legal marketing. There are no current approved INDs for Gerovital. In the past a firm called Fon-Amer Pharmaceuticals, Ltd., Las Vegas, Nevada, had two INDs in use which were limited to the treatment of mild depression. However, these INDs were withdrawn. Gerovital can be legally manufactured and sold within the state of Nevada.

KH3 is frequently accompanied by promotional literature or is labeled as a cure-all for such ailments as old age, premature graying of hair, wrinkling of skin, mental disorders, insomnia, decreased sex vigor, rheumatism, arthritis, heart problems, depression, etc.

KH3 frequently enters the United States through the mail and sometimes is labeled as "Free Trial Medical Samples."

Recently (within the past year or so), a firm called "The World Institute of Health, Inc." located in Walnut Creek, California, is sponsoring a pyramidlike sales scheme for the promotion and sale of Gerovital in the following three forms:

1. GH3
2. Zell H3
3. GH3 Cream

The institute employs sales people who act as

distributors and supply potential customers with promotional pamphlets and an order form. The customer then orders the product directly from the World Institute of Health, Inc., Grand Cayman, British West Indies via World Institute of Health, Inc., Walnut Creek, California.

A cosmetic company in Boston asked the Boston District to comment on a product called "Gerovital H3 Cold Cream" whose label promises to regenerate the skin, attenuate wrinkles, diminish senile efflorescence, and acne vulgaris. This is another variation which may be entering the country through legitimate entries, the mail, or in personal baggage.

In the past, there have been travel agencies that promote tours in KH3 or GH3 clinics in Romania. In many cases the agencies have informed their tour participants that they can bring back a year's supply of the product. Upon return to the United States, these people are having the drugs detained because of their new drug status.

GUIDANCE:

1. Continue to work with your local customs and post office officials advising them of all known ways of attempted entry of Gerovital, KH3, etc., including all the possible names and forms of the product and all known sources such as the World Institute of Health, etc.

2. Detain all products offered for entry as Gerovital, GH3, KH3, Zell H3, GH3 Cream, etc., on a "New Drug Charge."

3. Detain all commercial entries of the finished injectable and oral dosage form of Procaine Hydrochloride unless it is the subject of an approved NDA/ANDA.

4. Detain all bulk Procaine Hydrochloride

consignments unless they are being shipped to firms holding approved NDA/ANDAs or as otherwise permitted to obtain the drug for research, teaching, etc.

5. Detain bulk Procaine Hydrochloride consigned to drug brokers unless the consignee offers adequate assurance that the material is destined to firms or individuals holding approved NDS/ANDAs or are otherwise permitted to obtain the drug for research, teaching, etc.).

6. When you become aware of travel agencies promoting tours to KH3 clinics overseas, issue a letter to the travel agency telling them that they should advise their customers that KH3 is a new drug without an approved New Drug Application and is not permitted into the United States.

Alert No. 57-04 Revised
July 14, 1988
IMMUNO-AUGMENTATIVE THERAPY (IAT)
REASON FOR ALERT:

"Immuno-Augmentative Therapy" (I.A.T.), is a method of cancer management proposed by Lawrence Burton, Ph.D. The treatment is currently available at the Immunology Research Center, Ltd., Freeport, Grand Bahama Island, Bahamas, and in Germany. It has also been reported that Dr. Burton is planning to open clinics in Italy, Spain, Hong Kong, Singapore, Australia, Mexico, and Canada.

In December 1974, the Immunology Research Foundation, Inc., submitted an Investigational New Drug Application (IND) to the US Food and Drug Administration (FDA) seeking to initiate human investigational trials with I.A.T. agents. The IND application was placed in an FDA "inactive file" in March 1976. Following investigation of the Freeport Clinic in 1978, the National Cancer Institute reported that records were inadequate to evaluate I.A.T.

There have been legislative efforts at both the state and federal levels to legalize the use of I.A.T. In 1980, a federal bill failed, which was intended to exempt for five years the "blood fractions" used in I.A.T. from the requirements of the Federal Food, Drug, and Cosmetic Act. Similar lobbying efforts are currently being sponsored today by the I.A.T. Patients Associations. Laws were enacted in the states of Florida and Oklahoma that would have the effect of making I.A.T. agents available in those states. The Florida law was subsequently repealed.

Oklahoma required informed consent advising that the efficacy of I.A.T. is unproven.

The American Cancer Society has stated that it has found no scientific evidence supporting the claims that I.A.T. can prevent, detect, or predict the occurrence of cancer and none was found indicating I.A.T. is safe or effective for any or all types of cancer.

Dr. Burton has also been reported to use I.A.T. in the treatment of AIDS patients.

Dr. Burton claims that I.A.T. bolsters the deficient immune mechanism present in cancer victims with specific immune human serum fractions. He claims to determine the titer of "blocking protein," "tumor antibody," "tumor complement," and "deblocking protein" and then administers in one or a combination of the "immune substance" (except "blocking protein").

In 1984, CDC reported sixteen cases of injection site abscess formation experienced by patients of the clinic. One vial of each of the human serum protein injections, four in all, were examined for sterility by CDC. All were found nonsterile. Contaminants included species of staphylococcus, bacillus, Acinetobacer, and Moraxella-like organisms. In 1985, Washington State Laboratories tested eighteen vials of I.A.T. and reported that eight were positive for the HTLV-III antibody and all eighteen for the hepatitis B surface antigen (HBsAG). Confirmation samples tested by CDC demonstrated six of eighteen positive for HTLV-III and all eighteen positive for HBsAG. The presence of the HTLV-III antibody may indicate presence of the AIDS retrovirus. Over half of the seventy-two vials examined by NCI thus far have revealed these antibodies.

In July 1985, representatives of the Bahamas Ministry of Health, CDC, and the Pan-American Health Organization visited the clinic and determined that it constituted a public health hazard. The Ministry of Health ordered the clinic closed in July 1985; however, it subsequently reopened. We are not aware that any corrective actions were taken to preclude further direct hazards associated with contaminated I.A.T. agents.

A sample of Dr. Burton's Immuno-Augmentative Therapy frozen in a block of ice contained in a cooler was offered to FDA in Boston district during the summer of 1987. Boston district analyzed and found the product nonsterile. Biologics analyzed the AIDS and HG2 AB virus and found both negative. This is the only sample of I.A.T. that we have been able to collect since Dr. Burton cleaned up and reopened.

INSTRUCTIONS:

Due to the direct hazards that have been associated with I.A.T. and agents, all entries, whether in personal possession or mail, should be detained. Alert your local US customs and postal service officials informing them of the hazards involved with these products and the importance that extra efforts be made to cover mail imports and personal possessions of persons coming from these countries.

Alert No. 66-45
May 31, 1989
DIENNET FOOD SUPPLEMENT HERB DIET CAPSULES
REASON FOR ALERT:

Imported herb diet capsules called "Diennet Food Supplement," which were the creation of Dr. Marcel Diennet, who operated a diet clinic in Paris, France, were found to contain undeclared prescription drugs. A sample collected of the capsules and analyzed by LOS-DO confirmed the presence of undeclared diethylpropion HCL, diazepam, and chlordiazepoxide HCL at therapeutic levels. Dr. Diennet had admitted that he sometimes added drugs to his capsules. The Diennet Institute initiated a recall of their products in August 1988. Shipments of the diet capsules containing undeclared drugs appear to be continuing . . . automatically detain.

Alert No. 62-02
June 28, 1988
GERMANIUM PRODUCTS
REASON FOR ALERT:

Los Angeles and San Francisco districts have reported bulk lots of germanium sesquioxide being offered for entry into the United States from Japan. The product may be offered under such names as: Germanium Sesquioxide, Organic Germanium, GE-132, GE- OXY-132.

The products may be labeled for food or drug use. There are no approved new drug applications or food additives petitions for these products and there are no current INDs on file.

These products have been repacked as health foods or as OTC drugs with claims for use in such severe medical conditions as AIDS or cancer. Advertising literature has been identified which promotes germanium products for use in treating or preventing serious disease conditions under the following names: Germanium, Organic Germanium Sesquioxide, Pro-Oxygen, Immune multiple, GeOxy-132, Vitamin "O", Nutrigel 132, Germax.

INSTRUCTIONS:

Because these products are promoted as foods or as drugs, even if they are offered for entry as the bulk chemical (or in bulk dose form) without any labeling or claims, they should be detained using the food additive charge unless there is sufficient information to make the drug charge.

There are legitimate uses for germanium in the semiconductor industry. Therefore, if an importer shows that the intended use of the product is other than as a food or drug, the entry should be released with comment and appropriate follow-up should be made to assure the ultimate disposition is as indicated by the importer.

Alert No. 62-01 Revised
December 7, 1987
LAETRILE (AMYGDALIN)
REASON FOR ALERT:

During the spring of 1977, US District Judge Luther Bohanon (US District Court for the Western District of Oklahoma) issued a decision permitting the importation of Laetrile for the treatment of terminally ill cancer patients through a physician's affidavit system.

The decision providing for the affidavit system was reversed by the US Circuit Court of Appeals for the Tenth Circuit in December 1986. On March 24, 1987, Judge Bohanon issued an order ending the physician's affidavit system.

As a result, Laetrile is now handled like any other unapproved new drug product.

The generic name for Laetrile is amygdalin. However, it may be labeled with various other names such as madelonitrile, Vitamin B-17, amygdaloside.

Amygdalin is generally synthesized from the kernels of certain Rosaceae, which include apricots. Related glucosides include prunasin, sambunigrin, and prulaurasin.

GUIDANCE:

The importation of Laetrile (amygdalin) under a physician's affidavit is no longer permitted.

Alert No. 61-05
June 12, 1979
METHAPYRILENE
REASON FOR ALERT:

The agency has received three reports from the National Cancer Institute regarding the carcinogenicity (cancer-causing potential) of methapyrilene in rats. The agency has reviewed each of these reports and concurs with the conclusions reached by the Clearinghouse on Environmental Carcinogens that methapyrilene is a potent hepatocarcinogen in rats, and as such, a potential human hazard.

Methapyrilene is widely used as an ingredient in OTC and prescription systemic and topical human drug products, primarily in sedative sleep aids and allergy-antihistamines.

The known foreign producers of drugs containing methapyrilene are:

1. Loftus Bryan, Ltd., Rothdrum County Wicklow, Ireland (bulk methapyrilene fumarate).
2. Bolder, Ltd., 9 Immengasse 4004 Basle, Switzerland (bulk methapyrilene fumarate and bulk methapyrilene hydrochloride).

GUIDANCE:

Surveillance is indicated for imported drug products containing methapyrilene. If any are encountered, detain, charging: "The article is in violation of Section 801(a) (3) of the Food, Drug, and Cosmetic Act in that it appears to be a new drug without an approved new drug application (NDA) pursuant to Section 505 and appears to be misbranded under Section 502 of the Act."

Alert No. 60-02 Revised
June 21, 1988
ANABOLIC STEROIDS:

Anabolicum, Anadrol, Anatrofin, Asellacrin, Bolasterone, Bolfortan, Primotestin, Lipiodex, Curablon, Cyclofenil, Deca-Durabolin, Dianabol, Dihydrolone, Durateston, Dimethyzine, Esiclene, Equipoise, Exoboline, Finaject, Laurabolin, Crescormin, Proviron, Metanabol, Methandrostenolone, Nilevar, Nolvadex, Nondrabolin, Nor-Diethylin, Omnifin, Oxandrolone, Oxitosona, Parabolan, Primobolan, Quinalone, Stromba, Sustanon, Testoviron, Depot, Thiomucase, Triacana, Trophobolene, Uni-Test Susp, Undestor.

REASON FOR ALERT:

Steroids are being used outside of their approved indications by athletes to increase body size.

GUIDANCE:

Automatically detain all entries of human and veterinary anabolic steroids charging: "The article is subject to refusal of admission pursuant to Section 801(a) (3) in that it appears to be a new drug without an effective new drug application as required by Section 505(a) and appears to be misbranded within the meaning of Section 502."

INSTRUCTIONS:

Automatically detain if advised by CDER, Manufacturing Surveillance Branch, HFD-336, all entries of human and veterinary anabolic steroids.

REASON FOR ALERT:

Anabolic steroids may be safely administered under the care of a physician for replacement therapy in patients with hormone deficiency in males, and for certain gynecologic conditions and breast cancer in women. There are reports that the steroids are being used outside of their approved indications by athletes (without disease) to increase their body size.

There are reports that these steroids are being brought into this country and are being sold illegally. We are working with the Department of Justice and the Federal Bureau of Investigation to investigate reports of the misuse and illegal sale of anabolic steroids.

Alert No. 60-01 Revised
February 24, 1987
**TAGAMET (cimetidine) TABLETS FROM
 CANADA**
REASON FOR ALERT:

Minneapolis and Detroit Districts recently reported activity in the importation of Canadian Tagamet. Detroit district recently refused entry of a shipment of Canadian Tagamet which was consigned to Crosstown Drug, Hamlake, Minnesota. . . .

Smith, Kline & French Laboratories (USA) is concerned about such illegal importations and they are making every effort to stop them.

Smith, Kline, & French, Canada, Ltd., has not been implicated in the illegal importation. Two shippers that have been identified, Speedway Drugs, Edmonton, Alberta, Canada, and National Drug Ltd., Winnipeg, Manitoba, Canada, (shipper of product to Crosstown Drug) are wholesalers who do not purchase directly from the manufacturer but from other wholesalers.

Tagamet manufactured in Canada is considered a new drug which may only be imported/marketed in this country pursuant to an approved new drug application (NDA). No such approval has been granted, nor is any application for approval on file for the Canadian facility.

The unapproved product is produced by:
Smith, Kline, & French, Canada, Ltd.
1940 Argentina Road
Missisauga (Toronto), Ontario

The identifying features of the package are:

1) Generally packed in bottles of 1000 tablets;
2) The name of the manufacturer, Smith, Kline, & French, Canada Ltd., and directions for use appear on the label in English and French;
3) The label fails to bear an NDC number, nor is there an insert attached to the package;
4) The label bears a number required by the Canadian Government, known as a DIN number, which for Tagamet 300 milligram tablet is DIN #397474.
5) Tagamet (Canadian) is the same color, size, and shape as the American version, but the tablet markings are different.

While we have no information that there is any effort to import generic cimetidine manufactured in Canada, you should be aware that there are three Canadian manufacturers for the generic drug product, two of which have the same light green color as the American product. However, because of significant price differential, an attempt may be made to import the generic product. . . .

GUIDANCE:

Increased surveillance is indicated for SKF's Tagamet Tablets, (all strengths) and cimetidine tablets (all strengths) produced in Canada. If they are encountered, detain, charging:

"The article is violative within the meaning of section 801(a) (3) of the Federal Food, Drug, and Cosmetic Act in that it appears to be a new drug without an approved new drug application (NDA) pursuant to Section 505."

Alert No. 57-01
June 11, 1979 Revised
HUMAN PLASMA AND SERUM
REASON FOR ALERT:

Human blood and blood components are classified as biological products under the Public Health Service Act (42 U.S.C. 262). In addition, these human blood components may be subject to either drug or device regulation within the purview of the Federal Food, Drug, and Cosmetic Act. Section 502(a) of the Federal Food, Drug, and Cosmetic Act provides that ". . . A drug or device shall be deemed to be misbranded . . . If its labeling is false or misleading in any particular. . . ." Similarly, Section 351(b) of the Public Health Service Act prohibits the false labeling or marking of any package or container of any biological product such as human blood, plasma, or serum.

The two major sources of human blood plasma are: (1) plasma collected by plasmapheresis, i.e., Source Plasma (Human); (2) plasma obtained from expired units of Whole Blood (Human), i.e., Recovered Human Plasma.

In the past, the Bureau of Biologics has received allegations that human blood plasma and serum from hospitals and other clinical laboratories has been labeled "Reagent Use only" and exported out of the United States. This plasma-serum may be diverted for use in the manufacturing of injectable products in the foreign country or it may be shipped back into the United States as source material for injectable products. The Bureau of Biologics has also received allegations that human blood plasma has been imported into the United States for in-vitro use under the designation of "fruit juice" and "live tropical fish" among others.

GUIDANCE:

Alert local Customs of our interest in human blood and blood plasma or serum.

Source Plasma (Human) is a product subject to license and cannot be lawfully shipped interstate or imported into or exported from this country unless the collecting facility holds an unsuspended and unrevoked US license. Recovered human plasma, intended for further manufacture into licensed biological products, may be shipped interstate or internationally only under the short supply provisions prescribed by 21 CFR 601.22.

Alert No. 55-01
September 24, 1980
INTERFERON
REASON FOR ALERT:

During the past two years there has been increased interest and involvement of the medical-scientific community with the potential clinical applications for the product interferon. This increased activity has been supported, in part, by such organizations as the National Cancer Institute and the American Cancer Society. Clinical studies are being performed to determine, among other things, if interferon is effective for cancer treatment. Media coverage of interferon has followed suit behind the scientific community and provided the public with a large amount of information on the issue. A seven-page article in the March 31, 1980 edition of *Time* magazine is an example. Currently, most interferon is being produced outside the United States. Recently, at least one district office has encountered a lot of interferon being entered in the United States without either a license, or an IND or labeled in conformance with 21 CFR 312.9. In that instance a redelivery bond was secured. There are numerous other occasions when interferon may have entered the United States without any knowledge on the part of the agency.

The bureau perceives a great potential for misuse and consumer deception associated with interferon especially in the area of cancer treatment. In addition, because of its high monetary value the likelihood of other products being fraudulently misrepresented as interferon appears reasonable.

GUIDANCE:

Interferon, applicable to the prevention, treatment, or cure of diseases or injuries of man is a biological product subject to licensure pursuant to the Public Health Service Act Section 351, 42 U.S.C. 262(a), since it is analogous to a toxin or antitoxin.

Alert No. 62-04
May 18, 1983
VITAMIN B-15 (Pangamic Acid, Calcium Pangamate)
REASON FOR ALERT:

A product consisting of a mixture of calcium gluconate and dimethyl glycene, allegedly the "building blocks of Calcium Pangamate," salt of the so-called "Vitamin B-15," is currently being promoted as safe and effective for use in the cure, mitigation and/or treatment of a variety of diseases including heart disease, peripheral vascular disease, diabetes, cancer, liver disease, asthma, emphysema, arthritis, and alcoholism. There is no vitamin recognized as "Vitamin

B-15." Neither this so-called vitamin, nor any of its salts or precursors, have been by adequate and well-controlled studies to be safe and effective for any of these uses.

The Office of Drugs has received reports of attempts to import this product from Europe.

The final disposition of the Food Science Laboratories, Inc. case resulted in an order to condemnation and permanent injunction prohibiting Food Science Laboratories, Inc. from manufacturing, packing, labeling, or distributing pangamic acid products. The decision affirms FDA's contention that such products are adulterated within the meaning of Section 402(a)(2)(c), since they contain a food additive which is unsafe within the meaning of Section 409.

GUIDANCE:

When "Vitamin B-15" is offered for import as a drug, it should be detained charging," "801(a) (3)—the article is violative within the meaning of 801(a)(3) because it appears to be a new drug within the meaning of Section 201(p) without an effective New Drug Application pursuant to Section 505."

When this article is offered for import with no therapeutic claims it should be detained charging: "The article is violative within the meaning of 801(a) (3) in that is appears to be adulterated because it contains a food additive which is unsafe within the meaning of Section 409."

Alert No. 62-05
January 7, 1980
ALL STERILE INJECTABLE DRUG PRODUCTS
REASON FOR ALERT:

There is a need for injectable sterile quinine to treat Indochinese "boat people" who are infected with resistant malaria. The DOD has depot stocks from 1974 that were manufactured by Vitarine which FDA has tested and found acceptable for immediate use. However, there presently are no domestic producers of this dosage form of sterile injectable quinine.

The Communicable Disease Center (CDC) has identified three foreign firms as potential sources for sterile injectable quinine.

Since 1976, the FDA has insisted that domestic manufacturers assure the sterility of small volume injectables through process validation. We have openly stated that sterility cannot be assured through finished product testing; that only sterility of that portion of a sample tested by current techniques can be assured and that, unless the process being used has been demonstrated to be effective through validation, the manufacturer is not in compliance with CGMP, and the product is deemed adulterated under 501(a) (2).

Alert No. 62-06
November 24, 1980
DMSO (Dimethyl Sulfoxide)
REASON FOR ALERT:

DMSO is dimethyl sulfoxide, a solvent derived from wood, which has been the subject of considerable interest for its potential as a drug. Testing of DMSO as a drug began in the 1960s, but was halted in 1965 after experiments in animals indicated that it had adverse effects on the eyes. Experiments were resumed the following year with restrictions to be sure that patients were adequately protected.

At present, the only human use for which DMSO has been approved is for interstitial cystitis, a bladder condition. Testing of DMSO continues for other purposes, such as scleroderma, arthritic conditions of joints, tendonitis, and bursitis. Studies of DMSO for possible use in mental illness has been concluded with no evidence that it is effective for that purpose. No firm conclusions have yet been drawn about DMSO's usefulness in other conditions, such as spinal cord injuries and brain trauma.

It has been reported that industrial grade DMSO, devoid of drug labeling, is being used for self-treatment of arthritis and other disease conditions. The industrial grade product is not of the quality used for drug purposes and is not made under conditions that are necessary for the production of human drugs and protection of users. Side effects associated with its use include nausea, headache, and skin rash. Further, since DMSO is a "carrier" chemical, it could deliver harmful substances into the bloodstream or the skin if they are present in impure DMSO.

No foreign manufacturers of DMSO hold effective NDAs or INDs.

Alert local Customs of our interest in this product. If it appears that the product is consigned to firms other than those which might be distributors for a legitimate use, the product should be detained. . . . The article is violative . . . in that it appears to be new drug . . . (with) no approved new drug application.

Alert No. 66-01
December 1, 1975 Revised
CRUDE DRUGS AND PREPARED MEDICINES
    FROM THE ORIENT
REASON FOR ALERT:
FDA has found it necessary to give some attention to crude drugs and so-called "pre-

pared medicines'' imported from the Orient for use primarily by the Chinese population in the US. Due to increased trade, new sources for such imports can be expected from the Peoples Republic of China. With the probability of increases in drug imports from various China sources, it appears desirable that FDA give some coverage to the drugs, particularly as the labeling.

ACTION:

The Office of Compliance, Bureau of Drugs, suggests that as an initial action, districts contact the Importers of Record who have consistently dealt in the importation of such drugs from Formosa, Hong Kong, etc.

This is not intended as giving greatly increased attention to such importations; but is the opinion of the bureau that some tightening up of labeling should be undertaken for these drugs, and this would apply regardless of the country of origin.

Alert No. 66-02 Revised
April 21, 1977
GINSENG
REASON FOR ALERT:

Importers are continuing to offer for entry products containing ginseng. Some of these products have been labeled with medical claims and others have been represented for food use.

The Bureau of Drugs has informed us that they are unaware of any adequate scientific evidence or controlled scientific studies that demonstrate medical properties for ginseng, in fact, the *U.S. Dispensatory* dismissed the drug as therapeutically worthless and deleted it from its publication in 1950.

The Bureau of Foods has informed us that only pure whole, powdered, or ground ginseng used for the water infusion (the tea) is considered GRAS. The GRAS status of ginseng tea was based solely on human experience. All other food uses of ginseng must be covered by an effective food additive regulation or be affirmed as GRAD by an appropriate GRAS affirmation petition.

GUIDANCE:

Any ginseng offered for entry with medical claims would be regarded as a new drug and should be detained.

Alert No. 66-04
June 11, 1985 Revised
OIL OF EVENING PRIMROSE
REASON FOR ALERT:

Oil of Evening Primrose (gamma linolenic acid) is currently being promoted by some firms as a panacea for a wide range of conditions such as PMS, eczema, benign breast disease, obesity, alcoholism (cures damage done to brain by excessive drinking), and hyperactive children. The agency is unaware of any evidence to establish the safety and effectiveness for such claims.

FDA was recently informed by one firm, Efamol Research, Inc., Kentville, Nova Scotia, that they are conducting clinical trials with Oil of Evening Primrose and have approximately thirty US physicians working with them. To our knowledge, Efamol Research, Inc. has not submitted INDs for Oil of Evening Primrose. We are unaware of any domestic manufacturing of Oil of Evening Primrose and the article is being imported from Canada and England with either food or drug labeling. . . . Detain Oil of Evening

Primrose offered for entry . . . it cannot legally
be sold as a food or a drug except under the following conditions: (1) If sold as a drug, it is
considered a new drug and the responsible person must hold an approved New Drug Application (NDA); (2) If sold as a food, it is considered
a food additive and prior to marketing a food
additive petition must be submitted to FDA.

Alert No. 66-05
November 4, 1987
FOREIGN LABELED FINISHED DOSAGE
  PARENTERALS
REASON FOR ALERT:

Chicago District recently detained a shipment
of doxorubicin hydrochloride for injection in
finished dosage units labeled in English for the
United Kingdom. Entry was attempted under
the foreign manufacturer's (Faratalia) NDA
number, but that NDA only applied to a product
manufactured and labeled according to NDA
requirements. This article was purchased on the
world market, not directly from the manufacturer. Other shipments of various finished dosage parenterals had earlier been imported
labeled in a foreign language. CDB/Prescription
Drug Compliance Branch, Division of Drug
Labeling Compliance is concerned that such
products were not manufactured for marketing
in the United States and are not identical to the
NDA–approved product.

GUIDANCE:

Any parenteral drug product for human or
veterinary use, except antibiotics, bearing foreign language or non-US English labeling should
be detained.

Alert No. 66-06
March 1, 1985
HOMEOPATHIC CANCER DRUGS shipped by Erich Klemke
REASON FOR ALERT:

The articles are violated within the meaning of 801(a) (3) in that they appear to be new drugs without an approved New Drug Application.

Alert No. 66-08
January 12, 1979
DRUG PRODUCTS CONTAINING ADRENAL CORTEX EXTRACT OR ADRENAL CORTEX INJECTION
REASON FOR ALERT:

We have received the following information from the Bureau of Drugs:

For numerous years parenteral drugs containing adrenal cortex extract or adrenal cortex injection have been marketed with labeled indications for human use in the treatment of various conditions. There is, however, a lack of substantial evidence of these drugs' safety and effectiveness for their indications. The AMA Drug Evaluations, 1971 first edition, stated that adrenal cortex injection (adrenal cortex extract) is considered "an obsolete preparation for the treatment of adrenal cortical insufficiency." The *AMA Drug Evaluation*, 1973 second edition considers that "there is no known medical use for this drug." FDA's medical advisors concur that these drug products are not generally recognized as safe and effective for labeled indications for human use.

Therefore, parenteral drugs for human use containing adrenal cortex extract or adrenal cortex injection are considered as new drugs for which there have been no approved New Drug Applications.

GUIDANCE:

Detain all importations of parenteral drugs for human use containing adrenal cortex extract or adrenal cortex injection.

Alert No. 66-09
March 4, 1982
WOODWARD'S GRIPE WATER
REASON FOR ALERT:

Woodward's Gripe Water is promoted for infants including newborns and older children over twelve months of age and is labeled for gripes, acidity, flatulency, a quick and gentle way of relieving baby's hiccups, minor tummy upsets, and teething. The article contains, among other things, dill oil or dill water, sodium bicarbonate and 3.67 to 4.96 percent alcohol.

Woodward's Gripe Water is the product of W. Woodward, Ltd., London, England. It is also made by other companies throughout the world under franchises or other agreements with the main London, England, company or its affiliates. It has been used in various foreign countries for many years. However, in this country, it is not generally recognized as safe and effective for its intended uses, based on its formula and labeling, and therefore, is considered a new drug, which cannot be marketed without an approved New Drug Application. In addition, questions of safety have been raised by the Center for Drugs and Biologics, regarding the dill oil water ingredients.

GUIDANCE:

When Woodward's Gripe Water is offered for import by any firm, it should be detained.

Alert No. 66-10
July 1, 1983
"CHINESE HERBAL MEDICATIONS"
REASON FOR ALERT:

Chinese herbal medications have a history, dating back to 1974, of containing strong prescription drugs.

In 1974, four cases of agranulocytosis, resulting in the death of one person and extensive hospitalization of three others, were linked to use of these preparations. FDA analysis of the pills involved in the illness found phenylbutazone and aminopyrine, and other "herbal medications."

In 1980, several illnesses and another death were linked to the use of Chinese herbal medications, particularly *chuifong toukuwan*. Analysis of *chuifong toukuwan* from various sources found indomethacin, hydrochlorothiazide, chlordiazepoxide, lead, and cadmium.

More recently, in 1983, an additional brand of the *chuifong toukuwan* variety labeled only in Chinese (translated as product Number 13 below) has appeared in the Portland, Oregon, area. Trademark is a pair of concentric units surrounding a dragon intertwined about the numeral "7" (Seven Dragon Brand). The pills come sixty to a bag in a white plastic bag with a zip-lock closure. FDA analysis has found phenylbutazone at 10 to 18 milligrams per pill in the product.

None of the products list the drug substances

as ingredients. Investigation has shown that the pills originate from several sources, and usually enter the country via air mail shipments to health food stores, oriental food stores, novelty shops, and individual consumers. They are occasionally sold door-to-door.

Alert No. 66-12
April 15, 1981 Revised
GREEN LIPPED MUSSEL
REASON FOR ALERT:

San Francisco District first learned in 1976 that a product being promoted for the treatment of arthritis and sold as a food supplement was being offered for entry into the United States by the McFarlane Laboratories, Ltd., Auckland, New Zealand. The product, sold under the name of "Seaton" is made from an extract of green lipped mussel. The product was being promoted for use in the treatment of rheumatoid arthritis. The manufacturer in New Zealand indicated sales of three million capsules monthly in the United States.

Recently the Bureau of Drugs was informed that there is a group that is actively promoting the use of green lipped mussel extract for the treatment of arthritis.

Currently there is only one individual who has applied for an IND to begin clinical studies of this extract for the treatment of arthritis.

Alert No. 66-13
December 30, 1987
EAGLE BRAND MEDICATED OIL
REASON FOR ALERT:

During the past several years the subject product has been detained when it was encountered in import entries of Chinese medicines.

FDA has recently learned that the product has been reformulated. However, the old formulation of the product containing among other ingredients, 12 percent chloroform and 20 percent methyl salicylate, is being manufactured and supplied to other foreign countries. Under these circumstances, it is possible that the old formulation of the product may be offered for import into the United States. The product constitutes a consumer hazard in view of the carcinogenic nature of chloroform and its ban as a drug ingredient . . . and as a cosmetic ingredient . . . and because the product contains a high level of a potentially toxic ingredient, methyl salicylate, without bearing any warning statements required.

The new formulation of the product, which contains menthol (13.5 percent), ethyl alcohol (13 percent), methyl salicylate (4.5 percent), chlorophyll, mineral oil, and otto of roses and is offered for external use for relief of minor aches and pains of muscles, etc., would be acceptable for import on the firm's own responsibility pending completion of the OTC Drug Review.

Exclusive United States distributor for the new formulated Eagle Brand Medicated Oil manufactured by the Borden Company (PTE) Limited, of Singapore, is Anhing Corporation, Los

Angeles, California. The new formulated product is labeled on the carton with the statement "Anhing as sole agent." Entries by importers, other than Anhing Corporation, may be of the old formula and/or counterfeit product.

Alert No. 66-14
July 18, 1988
REIMPORTATION OF ALL PRESCRIPTION DRUGS FOR HUMAN USE
REASON FOR ALERT:
"The article is subject to a refusal of admission pursuant to Section 801(d) (1) in that it is a prescription drug manufactured in the US offered for import by other than the person who manufactured the drug and reimportation has not been authorized by the Secretary for use in a medical emergency as provided under Section 801(d) (2)." Under the provisions of subsection 801(d) (1), no one except "the person who manufactured the drug" may reimport an American-made prescription human drug.

Alert No. 66-15
February 18, 1988
PADMA 28 TABLETS
REASON FOR ALERT:
Padma 28 Tibetan Herbal Food Supplement ("Padma 28") is purported to be a combination of 223 herbs in tablet dosage form. The product is manufactured by Padma A.G., Zurich, Switzerland, and is imported into the United States by George Weissman, Inc., Padma Distribution Corporation, and Central Health Network which share a common tie. George Weissman has in fact stated that he holds exclusive rights to this product in North America.

Padma 28 enters the country without literature. However, oral and written claims for Padma 28 have subsequently been made by these companies. Specifically the product has been promoted for use in the improvement of cardiovascular circulation; reduction in levels of cholesterol and blood lipids; reduction of platelet aggregation; normalization of immunological responses; cure, mitigation, treatment, and prevention of atherosclerosis; bronchial asthma; skin allergies; acute and chronic viral and bacterial infections; peripheral arterial occlusion; hepatitis; angina pectoris; chronic coronary heart disease; hyperlipidemia; pyelitis; liver damage; hemorrhoids; upper belly syndrome; depression; impaired intellectual function; lethargy; myocarditis; pharyngitis; sinusitis; otitis media; bronchitis; pneumonia; and chest pains.

GUIDANCE:

Although slight variations in the label may be found, any product bearing the name Padma 28 should be considered the same drug. Please inform your local US Customs Service officials of our interest in these types of products, especially mail entries.

Alert No. 66-16
July 13, 1982
"STARCH-BLOCKERS"
REASON FOR ALERT:

A new line of products known as "Starch-Blockers" or alpha amylase inhibitions are being commercially marketed as a breakthrough in the field of weight-control management. These products claim to employ enzyme inhibition to block starch digestion and thereby have the effect of weight reduction.

Claims that "starch-blockers" affect the digestive function of the body cause them to be drugs within the meaning of Section 201(g) of the Food, Drug, and Cosmetic Act.

Because we are not aware of any substantial evidence which demonstrates that these products are generally recognized as safe and effective by qualified experts, "starch-blockers" are also regarded as new drugs under Section 201(p) of the Food, Drug, and Cosmetic Act. Therefore, these products must have approved New Drug Applications (NDAs) or they are in violation of Section 505(a) of the act.

Alert No. 66-17
April 3, 1987
"HERBAL MEDICATIONS"
REASON FOR ALERT:

There has been a marked increase in the importation of herbal products into the United States, especially from Asian and European countries. Our review of these products indicates that they include herbal teas, mixtures of herbs, vitamins and/or minerals and/or amino acids, etc., which are routinely labeled for the treatment of serious disease conditions (e.g., heart disease or cancer).

The Food and Drug Administration regards herbal products labeled for the cure, treatment, prevention, or mitigation of disease to be drugs as this term is defined in section 201(g) of the Federal Food, Drug, and Cosmetic Act. Also, in the absence of information that any of these products are recognized as safe and effective for their intended uses, we regard such products to be new drugs.

306

GUIDANCE:

We have little or no information concerning the composition of these products and the degree of hazard they may present to the consumer in the USA. Consequently, the districts should cover the importation of these products and when herbal-type products labeled for serious disease conditions are encountered, they should be detained.

Alert No. 66-20
January 31, 1986
"AZOQUE," "GRETA," "AZARCON," AND SIMILAR MEXICAN FOLK REMEDIES
REASON FOR ALERT:

The Food and Drug Administration received information from the California State Health Department that they had seized containers of a Mexican folk remedy called "Azoque" being offered for sale at a San Jose store specializing in Latin American imports. Other similar Mexican folk remedies called "Greta," "Azarcon," "Rueda," "Coral," "Alarcon," "Liga," and "Maria Luisa" were previously known to be offered for sale in the Hispanic communities throughout the US, predominantly among migrant workers in South Texas, California, and Florida.

These products reportedly are recommended for the treatment of *emphaco* (a general Spanish term for indigestion, diarrhea, and other stomach and intestinal illness) and are primarily given to infants and children. There is some adult use.

Azoque is the Spanish term for mercury, which is poisonous. Mercury and its salts are absorbed through the mucous membranes and are toxic, especially to persons exposed to them for extended periods of time. Azarcon and Greta are orange and yellow powders containing lead which pose significant hazards, especially to children. Greta, for example, is approximately 99 percent lead oxide. "Rueda," "Coral," "Alarcon," "Liga," and "Maria Luisa" are also believed to be lead-containing compounds. Use of these products may result in neurological disturbances including seizures, coma, and death.

GUIDANCE:

Detain, with analysis shipments of "Greta," etc.

Alert No. 66-11 Revised
August 31, 1983
"TATEX" TATTOO REMOVER
REASON FOR ALERT:

During 1976, three complaints of injury had been reported implicating this drug as the source of acute inflammation, cellulitis, and secondary infection of the skin.

All of the complainants indicated that the tattoo remover was received through the mail from the Atlanta Co., Pickering, Ontario, Canada.

During fiscal year 1982, there were two detentions of the product which were again received through the mail, indicating that it is still entering the country. The manufacturer/shipper was reported as the "Tatex Corp.," Pickering, Ontario, Canada. Detain all entries and mail entries of this product.

Alert No. 66-21
April 7, 1980
P2P OR PHENYL-2-PROPANONE (INGREDIENT OF METHAMPHETAMINE OR "SPEED")
REASON FOR ALERT:

The Drug Enforcement Administration (DEA), Philadelphia, PA, reported that P-2-P (phenyl-2-

propanone) from foreign countries is being smuggled into the US by criminal groups, such as the organization in Philadelphia from which DEA made one arrest and seized seven gallons of P-2-P on February 26, 1980.

P-2-P is the main precursor chemical used in the manufacture of methamphetamine (Speed). The chemical is a liquid usually bottled in one-gallon brown bottles. Its appearance is similar to urine and has a very unique and strong odor.

The tremendous number of clandestine laboratories which make Speed in the US have created a huge demand for P-2-P. Previously, the labs used the chemical supply houses and companies in the US as sources of supply for P-2-P, because they could order and possess the chemical legally. The only illegal substance was the finished product, methamphetamine (Speed).

On February 11, 1980, P-2-P was made a controlled substance pursuant to the Controlled Substances Act. This being the case, P-2-P must now be purchased from illegal sources by the clandestine laboratories.

Alert No. 66-22
November 4, 1981
"HOMEOPATHIC" DRUGS
REASON FOR ALERT:

FDA has reviewed the policy issues involved with the detention of homeopathic drugs for failure to bear the prescription legend and failure to bear the statement "For use only by or under the supervision of a licensed practitioner who is experienced in the use of and the administration of homeopathic drugs, and is familiar with the indications, effects, dosages, methods, and frequency of duration of such drugs."

Although FDA has, since the passage of the

Durham-Humphrey Amendment, stated in correspondence that homeopathic drugs should be restricted to prescription sale and labeled with the Rx legend, the agency has never actively attempted to enforce this requirement for domestic homeopathic drugs. We have, therefore, examined the issue from the standpoint of priorities, and we agree that homeopathic drugs of foreign origin should have the same enforcement priority as those of domestic origin. We have also examined the issue from the standpoint of the obligations of the US Government under the General Agreement on Trades and Tariffs (GATT). The GATT requires that imported products "be accorded treatment no less favorable than that accorded to like products of national origin with respect of all laws, regulations, and requirements affecting their internal sale, offering for sale, purchase, transportation distribution, or use." Although GATT does not prevent signatory countries from enforcing measures necessary to protect the public health, it requires that such measures not be "applied in a manner which would constitute a means of arbitrary or unjustifiable discrimination between countries where the same conditions prevail, or a disguised restriction on international trade." Thus, under the terms of this international agreement we cannot act solely against imported homeopathic drugs and leave the domestic products untouched.

The Bureau of Drugs will prepare a surveillance program to determine the current status of the domestic homeopathic industry (e.g., size, products, labeling claims) and the nature of the imported products. The information from that program will be used for an agency review of our policy on homeopathic drugs and for recommendations to the commissioner.

Until the commissioner makes a final decision on both the policy and the priority to be used for all homeopathic drugs, it is not appropriate to detain such imported drugs for failure to bear the prescription legend.

GUIDANCE:

Therefore, homeopathic drugs must be "released with comment" and not detained if they do not bear an Rx legend.

To avoid the problem of foreign shippers and importers using this change in enforcement posture as a means of entering various illegal drugs, check to assure that the article is recognized in the Official Homeopathic Pharmacopeia as a homeopathic drug. If the article is an official homeopathic drug and is in compliance with other applicable provisions of the act and regulations previously cited, but does not bear an Rx legend and/or does not contain the statement "for use only by or under the supervision of a licensed practitioner who is experienced in the use of and the administration of homeopathic drugs etc." the article should be "released with comment."

Alert No. 66-23
April 2, 1986
CATHA EDULIS (KHAT)
REASON FOR ALERT:

Catha edulis (khat) is a shrub cultivated for its leaves that act as a "stimulant narcotic" when chewed or used as a tea. (See below for scientific names and other terms used for khat.)

Its leaves and young shoots are chewed (or otherwise used by brewing a tea and smoking in water pipes according to the Drug Enforcement Administration) to get a stimulant effect, caused by the compound cathinone, which is similar to that of amphetamine and its congeners.

The issue of khat misuse was first raised at the international level in 1935 by the League of Nations when the Advisory Committee on the Traffic in Opium and Other Dangerous Drugs discussed two technical papers on this psychoactive plant. In 1957 and 1971, the commission on Narcotic Drugs recommended that the United National Narcotics Laboratory do research on the chemistry of khat. The World Health Organization (WHO) has also been involved with the issue of khat.

According to the Drug Enforcement Administration (DEA), khat is considered a drug of abuse in Ethiopia and some eastern African countries. DEA is concerned about the use of khat in this country, but was not aware of its entry. DEA cannot regulate khat because it is not on the "Controlled Substances List" at this time.

GUIDANCE:

Alert your local Customs office and USDA office of FDA's interest in preventing entry of khat so that we are informed of all such entries. . . . Detain all entries of khat.

SCIENTIFIC NAMES OR VARIANCE:

Catha edulis, Catha edulis Forskal, Catha Forskalii, Catha glauca comb. nov., Celestris edulis, Methyscophyllum glaucum.

COMMON NAMES OR TERMS:

Abyssinian tea, African tea, Arabian tea, Bushman's tea, cat, Catha, chafta, chat, ciat, crafta, djimma, flower of paradise, ikwa, ischott, iubulu, kaad, kafta, kat, khat, la salada, liss, liruti, mairongi, mandoma, maonj, marongi, mbungula mabwe, mdimamadzi, meongim, mfeike, mhulu, muirungi, mulungu, muraa, musitate, mutswari, matsawhari, mutsawhri, mwandama, mzengo, nangunge, ol meraa, ol neraa, qat, quat, salahin, seri, Somali tea, tohai, tohat, tsad, tschad, tschat, tshut, tumayot, waifo, warfi, warfo.

Alert No. 66-24
August 20, 1984
COLGATE DENTAL CREAM WITH DOUBLE
  FLUORIDE
REASON FOR ALERT:

Colgate Dental Cream is manufactured in England and Portugal with a double fluoride formula (0.76 percent sodium monofluorophosphate and 01 percent fluoride). Since a combination of two fluoride ingredients has not been marketed OTC in this country (the two ingredients may be used singularly in OTC toothpastes but not in combination) and the resulting level of fluoride is higher than is allowed in an anti-caries dentifrice, this product is considered an unapproved "new drug."

GUIDANCE:

When found, shipments of the above mentioned or similar products (other brands containing a double fluoride formula) should be detained.

Alert No. 66-25
August 10, 1988
MATOL
REASON FOR ALERT:

In 1984, Dr. Anthony Jurak and J.F. Bolduc formed Matol Botanical International Limited,

Montreal, Quebec, Canada, (aka. Snazz Corporation, 8006 East Jarry Ville De Anyou, Montreal, Quebec). MBIL manufactures a product called "Matol." Matol is a mineral preparation in a base prepared from extracts of flowers, foliage, roots, and bark of botanical plants. Matol was promoted through a multilevel marketing scheme for the treatment of ailments ranging from rheumatism of the spine to prostate cancer. The product never received widespread distribution in domestic (US) commerce.

Canada's Health Protection Branch (HPB) is familiar with Matol. The Drug Identification Number (DIN) of 652008 registered the product in Canada as a therapeutic mineral supplement. The HPN has taken regulatory action against the product based on certain advertisement claims. Canadian law only allows this product to advertise name, price, and net contents. The firm has now apparently complied with the Canadian regulations.

MBIL also manufactures a potassium mineral supplement called "Km." This product's labeling and formulation has been reviewed by the Center for Drug Evaluation and Research and has been found acceptable. Therefore the "Km" product is not subject to automatic detention under this alert. . . . When Matol is entered without labeling, charge "The article is violative within the meaning of 801(a) (3) in that it appears to be misbranded within the meaning of Section 502(f) (1) due to a lack of adequate directions for its intended use."

Alert No. 66-26
February 14, 1986
CU-7 INTRAUTERINE CONTRACEPTIVE
  DEVICE
REASON FOR ALERT:

The Food and Drug Administration has learned that an independent supplier is distributing counterfeit CU-7 intrauterine copper contraceptives.

CU-7 is an intrauterine contraceptive . . . (with) the approximate shape of the number 7. It includes a wrapping of copper wire around the vertical plastic limb of the contraceptive. Cu-7 has been classified by the agency as a drug because the copper wire contributes to the contraceptive properties of the product. The original manufacturer has recently announced they are discontinuing marketing of CU-7 because it is no longer profitable due to numerous lawsuits. However, they have not withdrawn the NDA for the product and therefore, the legitimate CU-7 can still be distributed. If counterfeit CU-7 is encountered, detain.

Alert No. 66-30
September 10, 1986
FOREIGN DIAL SOAP
REASON FOR ALERT:

Antibacterial soap marketed under the brand name "Dial" which has been manufactured in Cyprus, Korea, Canada, the Philippines, Mexico, and other foreign countries and is intended solely for use outside the US, is being diverted into the US at this time. Although the soap is produced by licensees of Armour International Company, the maker of Dial, the license does not authorize shipment into the US. As manufactured by the foreign licensees, the Dial does not comply with the United Stated Food, Drug, and Cosmetic laws and regulations.

All Dial soap is a drug under section 201(g) of the Food, Drug, and Cosmetic Act based upon therapeutic claims contained in its professional labeling, i.e., reduce nosocomial infections. Foreign Dial soap often does not contain the same quantitative or qualitative formulation of American Dial soap. In addition, foreign Dial soap is offered in the US under the Dial trade name and thus represents itself as American Dial soap when it is not. For these reasons it is an imitation drug.

Dial soap is also regulated as a cosmetic because of labeling claims as a deodorant soap. According to information received from Armour International, some of the foreign Dial soap contains illegal color additives. . . . Automatically detain all entries.

Alert No. 66-31
November 20, 1986
MINOXIDIL—RIVIXIL
REASON FOR ALERT:

As part of an IND study, the Upjohn Company is conducting clinical investigations to determine the effectiveness of minoxidil for hair growth. No other firms have approved INDs or NDAs for this drug's use for hair growth.

Under Drug Study Bulletin #285, issued April 10, 1985, regulatory action is being taken against domestic producers of minoxidil for hair growth.

As a result, bulk minoxidil powder was seized under charges of Section 505(1), 502(f) (1) and

502(a) . . . after being imported from ACIF Lits., Toronto, Canada, labeled for experimental use only. Audax was promoting the drug for commercial sale as a hair grower, but has since ceased importing or marketing it.

A minoxidil derivative, Rivixil, has been imported to hair salons for use in hair growth, The firm promotes Rivixil as a cosmetic, even though it is an unapproved new drug. Rivixil is believed to be manufactured by Kemyos Bio Medical Research, Binasco (Milan) Italy.

GUIDANCE:

Detain importations of minoxidil or related products when it is not imported by a holder of an approved NDA or IND.

Alert No. 66-34
December 10, 1986
ALL PRODUCTS CONTAINING
   CHLORAMPHENICOL PALMITATE
   MARKETED AS COMYCIN
REASON FOR ALERT:

The Food and Drug Administration (FDA) recently received a report from the New York State Office of Professional Discipline regarding the possible retail sale in Asian American communities of a product containing chloramphenicol palmitate for use by children.

FDA investigation, including sample collection and analysis, has confirmed the sale of a product containing chloramphenicol palmitate under the brand name of "Comycin Powder for Children" by at least one retail outlet in the Rochester, New York, vicinity. Comycin is distributed in individual envelopes with both foreign and English labeling which does list chloramphenicol palmitate as an ingredient and lists "Thailand'' as the country of origin. Label translation identified the manufacturer as Thai Chareon Bhaesaj (Comycin) Co., Ltd.

Chloramphenicol is a hazardous antibiotic that is clinically indicated only for certain specified serious infections and it should not be used in the treatment of trivial infections. The Center for Drugs and Biologics has confirmed that the use of chloramphenicol without the supervision of a physician would pose a potentially significant health hazard.

GUIDANCE:

Automatically detain without sampling all ''Comycin'' and other Asian products containing chloramphenicol palmitate or other chloramphenicol compounds as an ingredient and intended for retail sale.

Alert No. 66-35
February 11, 1987
REDOTEX AND OTHER DIET PILLS FROM MEXICO
REASON FOR ALERT:

Dallas district has reported that some clinics in Nuevo Laredo, Mexico, are engaged in the business of selling potentially dangerous combinations of otherwise possibly useful drug products to US citizens for weight loss.

According to newspaper accounts, the diet regimen consists of several drugs including diuretics, laxatives, thyroid hormone, depressants, and antihistamines. The primary drug associated with the diet regimen is called Redotex, manufactured by Medix, a Mexican pharmaceutical company. According to the Mexican equivalent of the *PDR*, each capsule of Redotex consists of the following:

318

- Tri-iodothyronine (*Triyodotironina*) 75 micrograms—a hormone used to increase the metabolic rate of tissues
- Norpseudoepinephrine (*Chlorhidrato de D-Norseudoefedrina*) 50 milligrams—an amphetaminelike drug
- Atropine sulfate (*Sulfate de Atropina*) .036 milligram—used as a respiratory and circulatory stimulant
- Aloin (*Aloina*) 16.2 milligrams—laxative
- Diazepam (*Diacepam*) 8 milligrams—a depressant (Valium).

Other drugs associated with or used in conjunction with Redotex include:

1) Ponderex 40, 40 milligram, manufactured by A.H. Robbins de Mexico.

2) Moduretic, manufactured by Merck, Sharpe & Dome de Mexico.

3) Asenlix, 30 milligram, manufactured by Grupo Russellsa—Mexican Pharmaceutical Company.

4) Ionamin, 142 milligram, manufactured by Pennwait Labs de Mexico.

5) Fluddro, Furosemide.

The products normally given to patients consist of Redotex and products number 1 and 2 listed above. Products 3 and 4 listed above have been reported to be substituted for Redotex in some instances. Newspaper accounts have also reported the occasional use of product 5.

A health hazard evaluation by CDB of the product Redotex has revealed that the use of Redotex poses a health hazard, especially when taken without adequate medical supervision.

The irrational combination of these thyroid, diuretic, stimulant, and tranquilizer drugs may cause serious and potentially fatal adverse reactions. These would include alteration of metabolic rate, increased heart rate, lowering or increasing of blood pressure, loss of body electrolytes by diuretic action, as well as confusion and hallucinatory states.

GUIDANCE:

Automatically detain.

Alert No. 66-36
April 9, 1987
HUMAN DRUGS CONTAINING DANTHRON
REASON FOR ALERT:

Effective March 28, 1987, danthron-containing products may no longer be marketed in the United States. Danthron is most often used in laxatives.

This decision was based on recent studies that chronic administration of high doses of danthron to rats and mice resulted in the development of intestinal and liver tumors and that danthron is, therefore, a potential cause of cancer in humans.

A. ACTION IN THE UNITED STATES:

The Food and Drug Administration has advised drug firms manufacturing laxatives containing the drug danthron to immediately discontinue their production and to recall them from retail store shelves.

Danthron toxicity in humans has not been specifically demonstrated but because of the potential risk, FDA has requested a halt to all manufacturing, relabeling, repacking, and further distribution in the United States of human drugs containing danthron as an ingredient.

. . . Detention is indicated on all (bulk, prescription, and OTC) articles of drug offered for human use that contain danthron.

Alert No. 66-37
June 28, 1988
EMERGENCY OTC OXYGEN UNITS
REASON FOR ALERT:

The Food and Drug Administration generally regards oxygen to be a prescription drug. Nevertheless, FDA recognizes that there are many circumstances under which it would be impractical to insist that oxygen be administered only under the supervision of a physician. Emergency oxygen units can be marketed for OTC use, but such equipment must deliver a minimum flow rate of 6 liters of oxygen per minute for a minimum of fifteen minutes (90 liters). Labeling for emergency oxygen for OTC use may not contain references to heart attacks, strokes, shock, or any other medical condition amenable to diagnosis or treatment only by a licensed practitioner.

Recently, small, OTC oxygen units imported from Japan have appeared on the market. Many of these OTC units are not suitable for any medical or emergency use and are being promoted for "recreational" use. Most of these units are incapable of supplying oxygen flow of at least 6 liters of oxygen U.S.P. per minute for at least fifteen minutes. These products are regarded as new drugs without approved New Drug Applications. . . . Detention is indicated on all entries of emergency oxygen units or other OTC units containing oxygen if they fail to bear the required labeling appropriate for their intended use and/or are incapable of supplying at least 6 liters of oxygen U.S.P. per minute for at least fifteen minutes.

Alert No. 66-38
June 8, 1988
SKIN CARE PRODUCTS LABELED AS "ANTI-AGING CREAMS"
REASON FOR ALERT:

Between April 17 and June 17, 1987, Regulatory Letters were sent to several manufacturers of skin care products that were labeled with exaggerated claims (e.g., reverses the aging process) that made the products unapproved new drugs. FDA believes that many of these manufacturers as well as other firms may be importing these skin care products with exaggerated claims.

An example of some of the claims that may render these products as drugs are that the product "counteracts," "retards," or "controls" aging or the aging process. Other claims that a product will "rejuvenate," "repair," or "restructure" the skin are also drug claims. A claim such as "molecules absorb and expand, exerting upward pressure to 'lift' wrinkles upward" is a claim for an inner structural change which would usually cause a product to be a drug.

INSTRUCTIONS:

All entries of skin care products should continue to be checked for drug claims until a district is convinced the firm's products are in compliance.

Alert No. 66-39
May 16, 1988
BULK PHARMACEUTICAL PRODUCTS FROM ROHM & HAAS, ITALY AND FRANCE
REASON FOR ALERT:

A domestic drug manufacturer has reported finding dichlorodiphenyldichlorethylene (DDE) and dichlorobenzophene (DCBP) in cholestyramine resin, a bulk drug substance. The drug substance is manufactured by Rohm & Haas, Mozzanica, Italy or Rohm & Haas, Chauny, France.

Cholestyramine resin, USP, is used as an adjunct to dietary therapy to decrease elevated serum cholesterol and low density lipoproteins (LDL) concentrations in the treatment of Type IIa and IIb hyperlipoproteinemia. DDE and DDBP are highly toxic chemicals with carcinogenic potential, and are usually found as the degradation by-products of agrochemicals.

Rohm & Haas, the manufacturer of cholestyramine resin, also known as Duolite AP143 and Amberlite IRP-276, is also a manufacturer of agrochemicals, ion-exchange resins, and acrylic emulsions. In addition to cholestyramine resin, pharmaceutical grade products, such as Polacrilin Potassium, a tablet disintegrant (Amberlite IRP-88), and USP Sodium Polystyrene Sulfonate, a bulk drug substance used in the treatment of hyperkalemia, are known to be manufactured. Other pharmaceutical grade products may also be manufactured in the plants identified above.

. . . Physically sample all lots of bulk pharmaceutical chemicals, finished drug products, and intermediate drug products manufactured by Rohm & Haas, Mozzanica, Italy, and Rohm &

Haas, Chauny, France. If contamination is found, detain the shipment.

Alert No. 66-40
June 20, 1988
SOME BULK ANTIBIOTICS FROM COPENHAGEN, TURKEY, FRANCE, ITALY
REASON FOR ALERT:

Foreign inspections of pharmaceutical manufacturers are being performed. FDA will detain affected products if inspection has revealed that a firm is not operating in conformity with current good manufacturing practices (GMPs). When and if FDA confirms that corrections have been made, the respective firm's pharmaceutical products will be removed from automatic detention:

1. Dumex Ltd., Copenhagen, Denmark: bulk sterile antibiotics
2. ANAS, Ismit, Turkey: bulk antibiotics
3. Compagnie Oris Industries Laboratory of Biomedical Imaging (aka LAPIB), Gif-sur-Yvette, Saclay, France: selenomethionine 75 injection
4. Instituto Biochimico Italiano Spa (I.B.I.) Milan, Italy, and I.B.I. Sud Spa (subsidiary firm) Aprilia, Italy: bulk and finished dosage form antibiotics.

Alert No. 66-41
March 2, 1989
UNAPPROVED NEW DRUGS PROMOTED IN UNITED STATES (REVISED)
REASON FOR ALERT:

The following products have met the criteria for automatic detention from all sources: adrenal cortex extract, adrenal cortex injection. It should also be noted that these products are also covered under Import Alert No. 66-08 "Drug Products Containing Adrenal Cortex Extract or Adrenal Cortex Injection."

Alert No. 66-43
December 6, 1988
ADRENAL CORTEX EXTRACT OR "THA"
REASON FOR ALERT:

Unapproved use of toxic investigational new drug. Although Alzheimer's disease is clearly a serious disease, the commissioner stated at a July 28, 1988 meeting that FDA would not exercise its discretion to allow patients to import "THA" for their personal use under the newly instituted mail import policy. That is because "THA" is known to be a potent hepatotoxin, and widespread exposure to the drug could result in many cases of serious liver injury. We have been advised by the Division of Neurological Drug Products that a problem exists in the recruitment of people for these active INDs because of the large amounts of "THA" currently being imported illegally.

The following is a list of other names under which the drug may be entering the country: tetrahydroaminoacridine, 1,2,3,4 tetrahydro-5 aminoacridine, 5-amino-1,2,3,4 tetrahydroacridine, Tacrine, Robotal.

Automatically detain all shipments.

Alert No. 66-44
March 23, 1989
CLOZARIL (CLOZAPINE)
REASON FOR ALERT:

The divisions of Neuropharmacological Drug Products (HFD-120) and Drug Labeling Compliance (HFD-313) reported that Clozapine (Clozaril) is being brought into the United States for personal use. Although the drug is the subject of a pending New Drug Application (NDA), it is not approved. Clozapine (Clozaril), a sedative, is associated with a number of serious adverse drug reactions, including agranulocytosis, seizure, hypothermia, and tachycardia; therefore, this product presents a health hazard and does not meet the criteria of the pilot guidance for release of mail importations. Detain all shipments.

Alert No. 66-B13
September 26, 1988
RU486

"RU486" or "Mifepristone" manufactured by Roussel Uclaf Laboratories, Paris, France, has been approved in France and in China. The drug is used to induce abortion and can be used up to forty-nine days after a woman's last menstrual period.

This drug will not be allowed entry under the "Pilot Guidance for Release of Mail Importations" which was issued July 20, 1988, because it does not meet the criteria in the policy statement.

Bibliography

Barnhart, Edward R. *Physicians' Desk Reference*, 42nd edition. New Jersey: Medical Economics Company, 1988.

Brecher, Edward M. *Licit and Illicit Drugs*. Boston: Little, Brown & Co., 1972.

Carey, John. "Why the FDA Needs a Miracle Drug." *Business Week*, February 19, 1989.

Clark, Cheryl. "In Tijuana, No Prescription Is Needed." *San Diego Union*, November 30, 1986.

Delaney, Martin. Project Inform Fact Sheets and Discussion Papers. *PI Perspective*, quarterly, 1988–1990.

"FDA Probing Generic Drugs." *The San Francisco Chronicle*, July 31, 1989.

Garrison, Jayne. "Compound Q Tests Serve as a Challenge to FDA." *The San Francisco Examiner*, July 2, 1989.

Gilman, Alfred Goodman; Goodman, Louis S.; Rall, Theodore W.; and Murad, Ferid. *The Pharmacological Basis of Therapeutics*, 7th edition, New York: Macmillan, 1985.

Grady, Denise, and Podolsky, Doug M. "FDA Allows Mail-Order of Foreign Drugs," *San Francisco Chronicle*, December 1988.

Griffith, Winter H., M.D. *Complete Guide to Prescription and Non-Prescription Drugs*. Los Angeles: Price, Stern, Sloan, Inc., 1989.

Guanino, Richard A. *New Drug Approval Process, Clinical and Regulatory Management*. New York: Marcel Dekker, Inc., 1987.

James, John S. Various issues, *AIDS Treatment News*, Box 411256, San Francisco, CA 94141.

Johnson, Otto. *The 1990 Information Please Almanac*. New York: Houghton Mifflin, 1990.

Kastrup, Erwin K. *Drug Facts and Comparisons*. 1989 edition, St. Louis: Lippincott, 1989.

Nielson, James Robert. *Handbook of Federal Drug Law*. Philadelphia: Lea & Febiger, 1986.

Payer, Lynn. "Rejuvenation Drugs." *Longevity*, June 1989.

Reed, Paul. "Daring to Stay Alive." *Bay Area Reporter*, December 3, 1987.

Reynolds, James E. F. *Martindale The Extra Pharmacopoeia*, 29th edition. London: The Pharmaceutical Press, 1989.

Seligmann, Jean. "At Last, Quicker Access to AIDS Drugs." *Newsweek*, July 10, 1989.

Shilts, Randy. "'HIV Consumerism' Punch Hits Kaiser." *The San Francisco Chronicle*, July 31, 1989.

——, "Secret AIDS Drug Tests Being Probed by FDA." *The San Francisco Chronicle*, June 28, 1989.

——, "Abortion Pill Endorsed by State Medical Group." *The San Francisco Chronicle*, March 7, 1990.

Silverman, Harold M. *The Pill Book Guide to Safe Drug Use*. New York: Bantam Books, 1989.

Simon, Gilbert I., and Silverman, Harold M. *The Pill Book: 3rd Edition*. New York: Bantam Books, 1989.

Stone, Brad. "FDA Talk Paper." Food and Drug Administration, July 27, 1988.

Waldholz, Michael. "Taking the Rx Out of Rx Drugs." *The Wall Street Journal*, June 5, 1989.

Warren, Sam. *Having Fun in Tijuana*. Warren Communications, San Diego, 1988.

Wright, John W. *The Universal Almanac*. Kansas City: Andrews and McMeel, 1990.

Index

332

Hiprex, 257; *see also* Hexamine hippurate

Histamine H$_2$ receptor antogonists: cimetidine, 90–92; famotidine, 99–100; ranitidine, 136

HIV: *See* AIDS

Homeopathic cancer drugs, 55, 299

"Homeopathic" drugs, 309–311

Hudson, Rock, xii

Human immunodeficiency virus: *See* AIDS

Hydrocortisone, 19, 21, 31, 106–107, 264; *see also* Timocort Hydrocortisone Cream

Hypertension treatment drugs: *See* Antihypertensive drugs

IAT: *See* Immuno-augmentative therapy

Ibuprofen: *See* Advil; Motrin

Ifosfamide, 198–199

Imipramine hydrochloride, 107–109; *see also* Tofranil

Immuno-augmentative therapy (IAT), 25, 42, 55, 280–283

Imodium, 253, 260; *see also* Loperamide hydrochloride

Import alerts, 54–56; abridged copies of, 269–326

Imuthiol: *See* DTC

Inderal, 261; *see also* Propranolol hydrochloride

Infertility drugs: cyclofenil, 189–190

Inosiplex, 199–200

Inositol niacinate, 200–201; *see also* Hexopal

Inositol nicotinate: *See* Hexopal; Inositol niacinate

Interactions, drug: *See* Drug interactions

Interferon, 55, 291–292

Intrauterine contraceptive devices, CU-7, 55, 315

Investigational drugs: *See* Drugs

Isosorbide dinitrate, 109–110; *see also* Pensordil; Sorbide nitrate

Isoxicam, 162–163

Isoxsuprine hydrochloride, 110–111; *see also* Duvadilan

Ispaghula husk: *See* Fybogel natural high fiber regimen

James, John S., x

John Bell & Croyden, 248, 267; sample price list, 267

Kefauver-Harris Amendment of 1962, 11

Kelfex, 251; *see also* Cephalexin

Ketorolac, 163

Ketotifen, 163–165; *see also* Zaditen

Ketotifen fumarate: *See* Ketotifen; Zaditen

KHAT: *See* Catha edulis

Laetrile, 5, 25, 55, 285

Lancet, 232

Lasix, 253, 259; *see also* Frusemide

Latamoxef disodium, 111–112

Laxatives: bisacodyl, 80–81; fybogel natural high fiber regimen, 103–104; sodium picosulfate, 139–140

Laxatol, 253; *see also* Sodium picosulfate

Levamisole hydrochloride, 201–202

Levomepromazine: *See* Nonzinan

L-5 hydroxytryptophan (L-5HTP), 165–166

L-5HTP: *See* L-5 hydroxytryptophan

Librium, 18; *see also* Chlordiazepoxide

338